The Anytime, Anywhere Exercise Book

**300+ quick and
easy exercises
you can do
whenever you want!**

*Enjoy!
Joan Price*

The Anytime, Anywhere Exercise Book

**300+ quick and
easy exercises
you can do
whenever you want!**

Joan Price, M.A.
with Lawrence Kassman,
M.D., F.A.C.E.P.

ASJA Press
New York   Bloomington   Shanghai

The Anytime, Anywhere Exercise Book
300+ quick and easy exercises you can do whenever you want!

ASJA Press
an imprint of iUniverse, Inc.

iUniverse books may be ordered through booksellers or by contacting:

iUniverse
1663 Liberty Drive
Bloomington, IN 47403
www.iuniverse.com
1-800-Authors (1-800-288-4677)

Because of the dynamic nature of the Internet, any Web addresses or links contained in this book may have changed since publication and may no longer be valid.

You should not undertake any diet/exercise regimen recommended in this book before consulting your personal physician. Neither the author nor the publisher shall be responsible or liable for any loss or damage allegedly arising as a consequence of your use or application of any information or suggestions contained in this book.

Icons created by Frank Rivera and included here by arrangement with Adams Media, Inc., an imprint of F & W Publications, Inc.

ISBN: 978-0-595-51478-6

Printed in the United States of America

*This book is dedicated to the special person
who spent countless hours listening to all my tales
and ideas: my dance partner and more, Robert J. Rice.*

—Joan Price

Foreword to 2008 reprint edition

The Anytime, Anywhere Exercise Book is even more relevant today than when it first came out in 2003. As a population, we're exercising less, not more, despite knowing how this impacts our health, energy, and appearance.

Only a few details date the book—we watch DVDs now instead of videotapes (Video Alarm Clock, p.31), and we listen to MP3 players and record onto digital recorders instead of audiotapes (p. 252, 255, 256, 258). Most airports no longer allow us to "stash carryon in a locker" (Terminal Workout, p.190) so we roll our carryon suitcase or wear our backpack while we powerwalk the airport.

Speaking of MP3 players, I'd like to add some bonus suggestions for using your iPod or other player to motivate and invigorate you as you do your *Anytime, Anywhere* exercises:

1. Create a playlist of up-tempo, motivating music from your music library and play it during indoor and outdoor activities. You'll feel peppier, move faster, and enjoy it more!

2. Download free workout music mixes in the style you enjoy and at the right tempo for running, walking, interval training, or dance. Do a search in iTunes or the digital music store you prefer for " podcast exercise music" and you'll be amazed at how many choices you'll find.

3. Download audio podcasts (and video, onto your computer) of Pilates, yoga, and other exercise classes so you always have a fresh routine.

4. Download non-music, audio podcasts on topics that interest you and listen as you exercise. I enjoy author readings and interviews, National Public Radio programs, and non-techie technology podcasts as I walk. The time flies, and I learn something new each time.

I applaud you for buying this book and resolving to incorporate "fitness minutes" into your daily life. I'd love to know how you fit these instant exercises into your schedule, and whether you've discovered new ones that you'd like to share. Please visit my website (www.joanprice.com) and email me (joan@joanprice.com) to let me know how this book is helping you reach your shape-up goals.

Enjoy your fitness minutes!

—Joan Price
April 2008

Contents

Acknowledgments

I am grateful to the many clients, students, and audiences who set me on the path to writing this book by telling me, "But I don't have time to exercise!" This is for you!

Many thanks to my agent, Linda Konner, for her steady and exceptional commitment to this project.

Thanks also to my consultant, Lawrence Kassman, M.D., F.A.C.E.P., for his expertise, warmth, and wit.

12

Chapter 1

9 # Introduction:
Why This Book
and How to Use It 3

6

You're Picking Up This Book for One of These Reasons . . .

- You're a busy person who doesn't have time to exercise. Between job and family, whatever spare time you can eke out of a day surely isn't going to be spent going nowhere on a treadmill.
- You exercise on weekends with a favorite sport or leisure activity, but that's it. That's all you have time to do.
- You're presently inactive. You don't have much stamina and cannot imagine yourself in a regular exercise program involving sustained workouts.
- You're overweight and haven't a clue how to find a physical

activity program that feels good, is safe for your body, and doesn't embarrass you by making you wear tights or shorts in public. Maybe you'd just better wait until you lose weight before starting an exercise program.

• You hate exercise. Being strong and slim would be nice, but not at the cost of lifting weights or huffing and puffing.

An hour at the gym? Laughable. A 30-minute walk or run? Forget it. A 45-minute aerobics class after work? No way. Any fitness program that demands big changes in the way you live your life or disrupts your schedule gets an emphatic "two thumbs down" from you.

Your solution: *The Anytime, Anywhere Exercise Book*, a collection of more than 300 exercises that fit into your day. Many take only 1 to 5 minutes apiece. Most of the longer ones can be done while doing something else. You can get healthy, fit, and shapely without adding any more hours to your day; and you can do these exercises at home, at work, in a hotel, or wherever you happen to be.

Fewer than 25 percent of American adults engage in even light-to-moderate physical activity for at least 30 minutes a day, the minimum recommended for health benefits. But fully two-thirds of the sedentary population would like to exercise regularly, if only they could get going and fit it into their lives. This book will show you how.

Our approach offers you a viable alternative that can improve your health, increase your energy level, and elevate your self-image and sense of well-being, just by becoming moderately active. You might find that once you start out on this program, you will discover how good it feels to be physically active and may eventually choose to take the next step: incorporating workouts that last 30 minutes or even 60 minutes (as recommended by the Institute of Medicine in 2002) into your daily life, most days of the week. If you do, you can lengthen and/or combine these mini-workouts into a longer exercise session. And of course you can use these quickie exercises as backups when life interferes with your workout schedule.

What You Will Gain from This Book

If you're among the more than 60 percent of adults who do not get the recommended 30 minutes of physical activity each day, let alone the 2002 recommended 60 minutes, don't be embarrassed—you're about to change that! If you're presently a nonexerciser or intermittent exerciser, you will find that getting your recommended 30 or even 60 minutes a day becomes easier, more attractive, and more realistic when you realize how you can accumulate "exercise minutes" in ways that are convenient, fun, and easy, while requiring an insignificant time expenditure. Instead of exercising for 30 or 60 minutes at once, you'll see how to accumulate those 30 minutes, a few at a time, throughout the day.

Can you really lose weight on this program? Absolutely! Look at it the other way around: You've likely *gained* weight by *not* incorporating short bouts of exercise into your daily life! Obesity in the United States has doubled in the past 30 years, yet we're not eating more food. Our modern life—with its labor-saving devices at work and home, parking places at the door of almost every destination, convenience foods, sedentary jobs, sedentary leisure activities (even for children!), and frantic pace—discourages us from most of the physical activity that used to be a normal part of life.

Look at all the possibilities for activity in your daily life where you now choose the "easy," inactive way. Now think about how you can choose the active way instead. That involves many quick, simple choices—like getting up to change the TV channel instead of using the remote and walking into the gas station to pay rather than paying at the pump—as well as choices that take a few more minutes, like taking the stairs instead of the elevator and parking a few minutes' walk from your destination. Researchers from the Cooper Institute in Dallas calculated that if you chose the active way to accomplish 20 simple, everyday activities, you would burn 8,800 calories a month more than someone who chose the sedentary way. You would burn 2½ pounds of body fat a month just by making these simple changes—that's 30 pounds in a year!

The Anytime, Anywhere Exercise Book is an immediate, practical aid for getting started and will become a well-read treasure the more you use it. If you're a busy person who can't fit exercise into your schedule, you'll see how you can incorporate activities that do not impact your time at all. If you're inactive, you'll find yourself taking your first steps toward fitness—and smiling through every step. If you have weight-loss goals, you'll discover how to burn extra calories through the course of the day without disrupting your schedule or even making time for exercise. You'll become more physically active, healthier, and fitter.

The other benefit of this book is that you get to make *choices*. This is a do-it-yourself, ever-changing program with you in charge. Boredom is a key reason that people abandon their exercise programs. But here you're mixing and matching your choices from more than 300 options and putting together your own, personal program that fits your lifestyle and preferences perfectly! If you want, you can develop a routine that you repeat week after week, or you can keep trying new activities and surprising your muscles and your mind. Variety is the spice of life, and you won't get bored using this book.

Why Short Bouts of Exercise Work

Remember those barking coaches, trainers, and instructors who insisted on keeping you moving for 20, 30, 45, 60 minutes, or 40 days and 40 nights (or so it seemed)? Exercise leaders used to think that if you didn't exercise for at least 20 to 30 minutes at a time, it wasn't worth doing at all. It turns out their information was incomplete. Although a full 30 minutes is ideal for getting a training effect, the benefits of exercise are not "all or nothing." Research scientists have discovered that you can get health and weight-loss benefits from *accumulating* about 30 minutes of physical activity each day. You don't have to get those 30 minutes all at once—you can get 10 minutes here, 5 minutes there, and so on, adding up to 30 minutes.

Why aim for a total of 30 minutes? A longevity study of 17,000 Harvard alumni published in the *New England Journal of Medicine* found that people who burned off approximately 2,000 calories per week through physical activity reaped the greatest benefits of longer life and decreased risk of disease. That's equivalent to 1 hour of moderate exercise 5 or 6 days a week (less time if you exercise more vigorously). But the researchers also found that although this amount of exercise is ideal, you get health benefits from *much less*. Burning about 700 calories per week—the equivalent of 30 minutes of moderate exercise, 4 times a week—starts yielding health benefits. Burning 1,000 calories a week (about 30 minutes of moderate exercise, 6 days a week) confers even more health benefits, especially disease-risk protection and increased longevity. The American Heart Association echoes this recommendation of 30 minutes of moderate exercise, most days each week. That's manageable, especially when you don't have to do it all at once.

And not doing it all at once is the key. The premise of *The Anytime, Anywhere Exercise Book* is that even a few minutes at a time of exercise "count" and can be fun and make you feel better. This is no gimmick. It is based on scientific evidence of the benefits of short bouts of regular exercise. Many research studies have demonstrated that brief sessions are beneficial to personal health and well-being, and this approach is one of those recommended by *The Surgeon General's Report on Physical Activity and Health* (1996). The health benefits of exercise kick in when you accumulate your 30 daily minutes of exercise, even in little bursts of a few minutes at a time, repeated many times over the course of the day and week. In weight management, for example, total calories burned per week are the key variable, not the length of time or the type of any one exercise session. Research shows that exercise in a number of short sessions enhances health, keeps the heart and lungs strong, helps with weight loss, and decreases the risk of premature death and a multitude of diseases related to lifestyle.

In 2002, the Institute of Medicine announced new guidelines promoting 60 minutes each day of moderately intense physical activity to prevent weight gain and achieve the full health benefits of exercise. While 60 minutes might be a praiseworthy goal—and achievable through our method of accumulating minutes of exercise throughout the day—30 minutes each day of moderate physical activity is still the recommendation of the American College of Sports Medicine, especially for people who are now inactive. Whether you aim for 30 or 60 minutes each day, the key is still short bursts of exercise that add up over the course of the day.

Short sessions can also be the key to sticking with an active lifestyle, especially for people who are busy or who think they don't like exercise. And it's fun to improvise by spotting and trying new ways to work a few more minutes of movement into your day!

Besides the long-term benefits of accumulating minutes of exercise in a variety of ways, the many short-term benefits will also appeal to you. Even 1 or 2 minutes of exercise at a time, done several times throughout the day, increases physical and mental energy immediately, enhances productivity, decreases stress and depression, and boosts your sense of well-being.

We are certainly not suggesting that a program of 1-minute-here, 5-minutes-there is the magic bullet for an optimal fitness program. We are suggesting that this approach is ideal for busy people—such as business people and mothers of young children—and others who do not exercise on a regular basis now. Also, our program provides a backup for people who do exercise on a regular basis, 30 minutes or more at a stretch, for those times when your regular schedule is topsy-turvy. It's a way to keep progressing during those days or weeks when work, holidays, travel, family, illness, or visitors make your regular program impossible.

Why Lifestyle Activity Works

Being inactive is hazardous to your health. Physically inactive people are almost twice as likely to develop coronary heart disease—the leading cause of death and disability in the United States—as are persons who get regular physical activity, according to *The Surgeon General's Call to Action to Prevent and Decrease Overweight and Obesity* (2001). Physical inactivity carries a health risk that is almost as high as cigarette smoking, high blood pressure, or high blood cholesterol.

If you're inactive now, you can change this without a giant life upheaval. The key is just to become more physically active in the course of a day, choosing the active way to accomplish something that you need to do anyway. Your activity doesn't even have to be what you think of as "exercise" as long as it's physically active. Lifestyle physical activity, such as walking, gardening, dancing, doing yard work, shoveling snow, taking the stairs instead of the elevator—in other words, behaving the way we used to, before life became so convenient and time-efficient—can be just as healthful as regular, structured exercise.

Moreover, this physical activity does not have to be intense or vigorous to bring you health benefits. According to *The Surgeon*

General's Report on Physical Activity and Health, regular *moderate* physical activity can substantially reduce the risk of developing or dying from heart disease, non-insulin-dependent (adult-onset) diabetes, colon cancer, and high blood pressure. This report recommends burning about 150 extra calories a day (or 1,000 calories per week) with moderate-intensity physical activities, such as walking, pushing a stroller, swimming, washing and waxing the car, dancing, or gardening.

How much do you have to do? It depends on the intensity of the exercise. More intense requires shorter time; less intense requires longer time. For example, burning 150 calories might take 15 minutes of swimming laps, 30 minutes of walking briskly, or 45 minutes of washing and waxing the car. That's approximate, depending also on your weight and how vigorously you're doing the activity.

How the Book Is Organized and How to Use It . . .

The Anytime, Anywhere Exercise Book describes quick aerobic, strengthening, and stretching activities, organized by a variety of locations in which they can be done: home, park, office, airport, or hotel, for example. We include exercises that you can do while you wait for something: a bus, a slow-loading Web page, or a barely moving post office line, for instance. We have exercises you can do while talking on the phone, cooking, driving, showering, shopping, and doing a variety of other everyday activities. We have exercises that you can do anytime, anywhere that work and stretch your muscles and help get you to your fitness goals. These are also tension-relievers, ideal when a hectic day threatens to leave you stressed and aching.

You can find a new activity instantly that you can try for 1 minute or more that fits where you are or what you are doing at many times during the day. These activities are both fun and beneficial to mental and physical health. The exercises in the book are grouped mostly by the physical location in which each can be effectively done.

Two keys to sticking to an exercise program are variety and convenience. *The Anytime, Anywhere Exercise Book* has both: many different exercises that can be done wherever you are and that fit into whatever time you have available, even if it's only 1 or 2 minutes.

And this book goes beyond just the exercises. Sticking with a program of physical activity, even in this easy-to-find-the-time way of doing it, requires more than just descriptions of easy-to-do, easy-to-fit-in mini-workouts. You also need advice on the "mind-stuff" of getting motivated, how to get started the right way, how to stick with it, and how to make exercise fun. You also need advice about such practical matters as using proper technique, choosing equipment, and staying safe. We provide a variety of tips on these subjects, too, in the "Getting It Together" chapters organized by topic, separated from the exercise chapters. Here's where you can gain the mental tools for becoming a physically active person, as well as the nuts and bolts of creating and maintaining a program that you'll find satisfying and will get you to your goals.

You can either choose a "Getting It Together" category or an exercise location that fits your needs at the moment, or open at random and find appealing exercises to do and interesting tips to read. Have fun with this book—skim, read, and try an assortment of activities. Out of our 300-plus exercises, you'll find a variety that feel great, make sense to you, fit your lifestyle, and you find enjoyable. That's what lifestyle exercise is all about!

What Do the Icons Mean?

All of the exercises have icons. This way, if you want to find, say, stretches you can do at work, you can find them at a glance.

AEROBIC/CARDIO: indicates that an exercise is aerobic or cardiovascular (meaning that it raises your heart rate and conditions your heart and lungs).

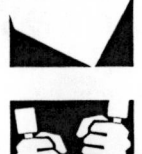
MUSCLE/STRENGTH: indicates muscle strengthening using resistance.

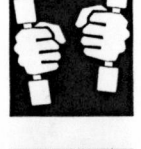
STRETCH/FLEXIBILITY: indicates stretching or flexibility (meaning that the exercise relaxes your muscles and helps you become more limber).

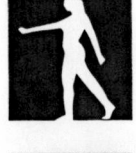
DYNA-BANDS: Dyna-Band icons, which mean that the exercises can be done with Dyna-Bands, Therabands, surgical tubing, or other resistance-weight, stretchy, exercise tools. (See the Resources Appendix for more information.)

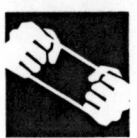
EXERCISE: indicates that an exercise is too light an intensity to qualify as aerobic or muscle strengthening, but still counts as valuable physical activity and is worth doing. Or the icon might indicate a list of activities that cross different categories.

As you try our exercises, you'll undoubtedly find some especially appealing, and you'll also discover and invent activities of your own. We'd love to hear about your experiences using this book, your discoveries, and your ideas for additional exercises. Please e-mail these to Joan Price at *joan@joanprice.com*.

12

Chapter 2

9   **Getting It Together: Starting Right**   3

6

T HE GOOD NEWS about starting to incorporate more physical activity into your life is that simply changing from inactive to moderately active yields dramatic health, fitness, and weight-loss benefits. If you've been inactive, these tips will help you make this change safely and comfortably and will help you prepare your mind as well as your body for this transition.

In a Nutshell

You don't need to be a sweat-driven, committed exerciser to get healthier and fitter. You do need to make a change in the amount **15** of physical activity you do on a regular basis. According to *Physical Activity and Health: A Report of the Surgeon General*, this is the bottom line:

- People who are usually inactive can improve their health and well-being by becoming even moderately active on a regular basis.
- Physical activity need not be strenuous to achieve health benefits.
- Greater health benefits can be achieved by increasing the amount (duration, frequency, or intensity) of physical activity.

Start Slowly

It's tempting, now that you've made the decision to increase your physical activity, to jump right in and choose six exercises from one chapter, ten from another chapter, and so on—and that's just for Day One. If you start out like wildfire, you're likely to burn out quickly and abandon your program. A better approach, if you've been inactive, is to start slowly and intentionally and gradually build up your physical activity to your goal amount. This helps to give your body time to adjust and avoid the soreness and injury risk that comes with doing too much, too fast, too soon. It also gives your mind a chance to adjust and accept your new changes.

Don't rush to do it all at once. Realize that if this approach to exercise works for you, you've got the rest of your life to practice it. And if it works, you've probably got more life—and quality of life!—ahead of you than you would have had otherwise! If you start gradually, you will be more likely to enjoy exercising, *and* you will be able to stay with it. Above all, enjoy your workouts, even (especially!) when they barely take 1 minute.

Make a Plan

Leaf through this book, concentrating on the chapters that fit your schedule this week. Choose some easy, enjoyable exercises to start with. Pick out four or five that you think you will *really enjoy* doing the first day and that fit your schedule. Maybe you'll choose one exercise that you can do first thing in the morning, a couple to do at work, and one to do at home in the evening. The next day, keep your favorites and try two or three new ones. Keep repeating your favorites and adding new ones through the week. Choose one longer activity for the weekend that can double as an enjoyable, social time with friends or family or a welcome, solitary retreat.

The next week, add or substitute a few different activities, and try something new on the weekend. And so on, until you're accumulating 30 minutes or more of physical activity a day. This might take weeks or it might take months. The point is to make movement fun, because that's what will help you stick to it.

As you progress, keep incorporating the activities that are the most enjoyable, and experiment with new ones that intrigue you. As you try different activities, flag your favorites and mark up the book with your comments. Months down the road, you might find you've created a routine that works for you, or you might still enjoy the variety of trying new activities. With more than 300 options, you won't run out of possibilities!

=========== **Benefits of Physical Activity** ===========

You know that exercise is good for you, but do you know how good? If you get regular physical activity most days of the week, your health improves in the following ways, according to *Physical Activity and Health: A Report of the Surgeon General*:

- Reduces the risk of dying prematurely (from all reasons, including accident).
- Reduces the risk of dying from heart disease.
- Reduces the risk of developing diabetes.
- Reduces the risk of developing high blood pressure.
- Helps reduce blood pressure in people who already have high blood pressure.
- Reduces the risk of developing colon cancer.
- Reduces feelings of depression and anxiety.
- Helps control weight.
- Helps build and maintain healthy bones, muscles, and joints.
- Helps older adults become stronger and better able to move about without falling.
- Promotes psychological well-being.

The Components of Fitness

There are three main components of fitness that complement each other and give you a balanced program. When you're just starting out, don't worry too much about how much you do of each, but do try to incorporate all three in your program.

- Aerobic—also known as **cardiovascular**—exercise uses your large muscles (such as your legs, thighs, and back) in a rhythmic manner to raise your heart rate and keep it elevated for a period of time. You can get a heart-rate monitor to know exactly how high your heart rate is, aiming for 60 to 85 percent of 220-minus-your-age, or you can usually judge it in this easy way: You're aerobic when you're breathing faster, feeling warmer, and breaking a sweat, but you're not gasping. You can still talk in full sentences. Aerobic literally means "with oxygen." Aerobic exercise increases the amount of oxygen that is delivered to your muscles, improving stamina and endurance and conditioning your heart and lungs. Aerobic exercise demands a higher expenditure of calories, so it burns stored fat. Examples of aerobic exercise are brisk walking, bicycling, jogging, skating, swimming, rowing, and cross-country skiing. Lifestyle activities can be aerobic, also, if they are vigorous, such as climbing stairs, fast vacuuming, fast dancing, mopping, mowing with a hand mower, digging in the garden, and raking leaves.

- **Strength training**—also known as **muscle strengthening or resistance training**—makes your muscles work harder than usual against resistance—something you push, pull, or lift, such as weights, machines, bands, tubing, or sometimes body weight—so they get stronger. Stronger muscles not only help you lift and carry heavier things, they help you avoid injury, give you shapely definition and a more youthful appearance, help to keep your bones strong, and burn calories faster. Realize that if you don't strengthen your muscles, they don't stay the same—they weaken as you get older. Combat that with strength training, so you get stronger instead of weaker.

- **Stretching**—also known as **flexibility training**—lengthens and relaxes your muscles. In normal activity and especially during exercise, we contract (shorten) our muscles as we work them. Leaving the muscles contracted is likely to lead to muscle tightness, fatigue, soreness, and, eventually, decreased flexibility. Stretching regularly, however, loosens and lengthens the muscles, increases range of motion, and relieves stress. Definitely stretch immediately after aerobic or strength exercise. You might also find it helpful to wake up your muscles in the morning with stretching and to stretch tired or tense muscles throughout the day.

Your Own Pace

If you're just starting a fitness program, don't worry too much about getting your heart rate up. In fact, you might have to be careful *not* to let it get too high. If you're out of breath, gasping, feeling light-headed, or unable to talk, you're exercising at too high an intensity for your fitness level. Slow down. Take breaks. Never push through discomfort or shortness of breath. Don't try to keep up with someone moving more quickly than is comfortable for you. Realize that you *will* improve steadily, and don't be impatient. Honor your own level and your new commitment to getting in shape.

Easing into Exercise

Some experts say it takes 3 to 6 months to make exercise a habit. People who stick to a fitness program past 6 months tend to make a lifetime commitment. They may have lapses, but they come back to it. That's because they've trained their minds and bodies to expect exercise, and they've experienced the immediate benefits, such as increased energy, decreased stress, and a sense of well-being. They like the way they feel and look, and they're more alert and productive. It's no longer difficult—in fact, they feel better when they *do* exercise than when they don't. Their quality of life is enhanced.

But when you're first starting out, it feels difficult, both physically and mentally. How do you stick to it while it's a struggle?

Start by doing *some* easy physical activity on a regular basis. This book is a great solution, because you're doing many short bursts of activity, just a little at a time, training your body and mind to expect it frequently. Do what's comfortable—no pain, all gain. For you, that might be 10 minutes a day at first, or it might be 5 minutes.

Get to know your body. At first, do a little less than you think you can to see how you feel later and the next day. Then, when you're feeling used to the activity, start pushing gently to do just a little more. There's no rush to work up to the health goal of 30 (or 60, depending on which guidelines you follow) minutes a day—you're getting stronger every day that you're physically active, and this will make it easier to add minutes when you're ready. Stay tuned to how you feel, physically and mentally, both during exercise and afterwards.

Consistency will get you over the hump. Your mind and body will adjust. You know you're there when you realize you feel better when you do exercise than when you don't!

Realize that you're not in competition with anyone except the you of yesterday. It took many years to put on that extra weight or gradually lose your muscle tone—you won't be changing that overnight. This isn't something you're doing just until the class reunion or swimsuit season. This is a lifetime commitment, so give yourself permission to take it slowly.

=== **A Lapse Isn't a Relapse** ===

If you fall off the exercise wagon, get up and try it again. Professional figure skater Scott Hamilton fell on the ice during his first performance coming back after testicular cancer surgery. "It's okay!" he said with a grin. "You can't succeed unless you're willing to fail. You can't land it unless you try it."

Calories Out

If your object is to lose weight, realize that increasing your physical activity will benefit you in several ways. First, you burn more calories exercising than not exercising, sometimes five to seven times more. As long as you don't eat more to compensate, these extra calories burned will start to come off your body fat. But the weight-loss benefits don't stop there: Exercising also raises your resting metabolic rate—the rate at which you burn calories at rest—so you burn more calories even when you stop. Further, you gain muscle, which is metabolically active. That means that muscle requires more energy (calories) simply to maintain itself, so you're burning still more calories just feeding your hungry muscles.

Scale Savvy

Speaking of muscles, realize that muscle weighs more than fat, although it's denser and therefore makes you look slimmer.

Imagine the difference between a plateful of chicken fat and a plateful of muscled chicken thigh. The fat is bigger and fluffier (okay, *fatter!*), but the obviously "thinner" thigh weighs more. See the point? So at first, as you're losing body fat and gaining muscle, your scale won't know the difference—it doesn't know it's weighing that slim muscle tissue instead of that fluffy fat, and it might show you a weight that discourages you. So track your progress with a tape measure instead—when you see that you're losing inches, you know you're losing body fat. It may take a while before your progress shows on the scale, but research shows that exercise is the strongest predictor of long-term success in weight management.

=========== **Should You See Your Doc?** ===========

If you've been inactive, it's wise to consult your physician before starting an exercise program if you fit any of the following categories:

- You have or are at risk for heart disease.
- You have chest pain, pressure in the chest, or shortness of breath when you exert yourself.
- You have a history of lung disease.
- You have or are at risk for diabetes.
- You have a bone or joint condition or limitation that affects your capacity for physical activity.
- You are obese.

- You are a man over age 40 planning a new, vigorous physical activity program.
- You are a woman over age 50 planning a new, vigorous physical activity program.
- You have high serum cholesterol.
- You have high blood pressure.
- You smoke cigarettes.
- You abuse drugs or alcohol.
- You take prescription medications.

When your physician tells you, "Go for it!" (which is likely, because physical activity helps most of these conditions), be sure you start out slowly and gradually. Stay aware of how you feel during and after physical activity.

12

Chapter 3

9   **At Home: By the Dawn's Early Light**   3

6

WHETHER OR NOT you see yourself as a morning exerciser, you can accumulate 5 to 30 minutes of exercise at the beginning of the day with a minimum of effort and just a little planning. The advantages are many: All day long, you'll have more energy, a spring in your step, a sharper mind that can increase mental productivity, and a feeling of well-being. An added benefit is that the day's stress won't get to you as much. Exercise is like taking an energy-plus-calming pill with no side effects!

Bed Back Stretch. Here's one exercise you can do before getting out of bed. Lie on your back with the left leg stretched out straight on the bed and the right leg bent, right thigh pulled in toward your chest, hands behind the thigh or knee. Relax, letting the lower back stretch comfortably. Then change sides. If it feels good, bring both thighs in toward the chest, hands behind the thighs or knees.

Calves with Teeth. Do leg raises while you brush your teeth. Stand on a phone book (the bigger the better), toes toward the book's spine, your heels hanging over the edge opposite the spine. Push up onto the balls of your feet for 2 seconds, hold in that position for 2 seconds, then let yourself down again for 4 seconds. Tighten your abdominals and buttocks to aid in balance, and keep your back in a neutral position (that is, don't lean either forward or back). If you need help balancing, lightly touch the sink while you do the exercise, but try not to lean on the sink. Don't rush! Repeat until you've brushed for the full 2 minutes that dentists recommend or until your calves are tired, whichever comes first. This exercise strengthens the lower legs and also works the abdominals and back if you stand up straight and don't grip the sink. If the phone book feels too unsteady, take your toothbrush with you and do this exercise on the lower step of a staircase.

Advanced Calves. Do the above exercise on one leg at a time. Stand with your right foot on the phone book, the left leg bent, the top of the left foot pressing against the right calf. Do the leg raises balancing on one leg for 8 slow repetitions, then switch legs. You'll work the abdominals and back postural muscles and train your balance skills in addition to working the calves.

Cardio Alarm Clock. Instead of hitting the snooze button, energize yourself with 5 to 20 minutes of aerobic exercise in the morning. If you have cardio equipment (exercise bike, treadmill, rower, aerobic rider, stepper), get on it while the coffee's brewing, and watch the early news. Make sure your equipment is in a spot that's convenient, but, especially if you live with other people, not in their way—a difficult but not impossible task if you put your mind to it!

Thigh Flossing. Do the Phantom Chair (a.k.a. "wall sit") while you floss your teeth: Stand with your back against a wall, and slowly slide partway down, keeping your back in contact with the wall. Walk your feet away from the wall, making sure they stay right under your knees, until your thighs are taking your weight and you look like you're sitting in an invisible chair. Hold that pose, breathing normally, until your thighs scream, "Enough!" This is a great thigh strengthener.

 **Coffee Jog.** If you can't do a thing until your first sip of coffee, jog (instead of lurch) to the kitchen, and jog—in place or traveling—while you're doing your coffee ritual: grinding beans (or opening the ground coffee), getting your favorite mug, and so on. A 150-pound person burns 9 calories per minute jogging in place.

What About Eating?

How do you time your exercise minutes with breakfast? It's best not to exercise on a full stomach—your body doesn't like trying to digest and exercise at the same time—so plan your workout minutes before breakfast. If you get too hungry or dizzy when you exercise without eating, have a small snack such as a banana, slice of bread, or glass of orange juice to fuel your workout. Then follow your activity with a nutritious breakfast.

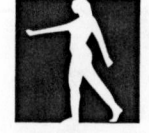 **Gentle Wake-Up Call.** If the idea of an early-morning cardio workout makes you pull the covers over your head, how about a calming yoga or tai chi wake-up, or a gentle stretch? If you're experienced, do your own gentle workout. If you'd like a leader, choose from several excellent videotapes. (Read Chapter 9 and the Resources Appendix before you buy.)

The Anytime, Anywhere Exercise Book

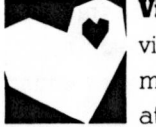 **Video Alarm Clock.** Get a couple of aerobic exercise videotapes, and have one ready to go first thing in the morning. Don't ask yourself if you feel like exercising at this cruel hour—just do it in your jammies. Even if you only have time for 5 minutes, it will rev up your energy and burn calories, especially if your choice is aerobic dance, step, or cardio kickboxing. A 150-pound person burns 6 to 8 calories per minute with aerobic dance, depending on impact and intensity, and 9 to 12 calories per minute with step aerobics, depending on step height, according to the American College of Sports Medicine. (Read Chapter 9 for information about choosing and using exercise videos, and see the Resources Appendix for suggestions about where to order them.)

Jump Out of Bed. Warm up by bustling around the house a bit, then pull out your jump rope for a 5- to 10-minute energizer. Take at least 2 minutes to work up to speed gradually before full-out jumping. Then stay at a pace that gets your heart rate up, but doesn't make you gasp. Use the last 60 to 90 seconds to cool down by gradually slowing your pace. Try to leave time for a stretch afterwards. A 150-pound person burns from 9 to 14 calories per minute jumping rope, depending on speed. If you don't have the stamina for rope jumping, try rope skipping instead. (You don't have a jump rope? Just skip!)

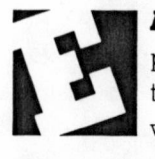 **Active Bed Making.** Walk around the bed as much as possible when you make the bed. Also stretch across the bed to smooth corners rather than just smoothing what's closest to you. Every bit of activity counts!

Dance Yourself Awake. Play your favorite, fast-paced music first thing in the morning, and dance around the house. We don't care (although your roommates might!) whether it's techno, swing, hip-hop, Viennese waltz, or country two-step, as long as it gets your feet moving and puts a smile on your face.

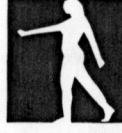 **After-Cardio Stretch.** Whichever cardio wake-up you use, stretch the lower body afterwards with this sequence:

1. Stand facing a wall, pushing against it with both hands. Step back with the right leg and press the right heel down. The left leg is slightly bent. Feel the stretch in the right calf.
2. Then bring the right leg forward a couple of inches and slightly bend the right knee, feeling the stretch go lower in the calf. Repeat steps 1 and 2 with the left leg.
3. Stand upright, facing the wall, touching it with your left hand for balance. Reach back with the right hand and,

keeping the thighs together, bend the right knee until you can hold on to your right ankle (or sock or pant leg) behind you. Try to keep your thighs together and your back straight. You'll feel the stretch in the right quadriceps (front of the thigh). Repeat with the left leg.

4. Step back with the right leg. Align the left knee over the ankle and slide the right leg back until you sink into a comfortable lunge, left thigh parallel to the floor. The right knee is bent (a little or a lot, depending on your comfort), and the right heel is off the ground. Go only to the point of comfort, and don't let the left knee go forward of the foot. Your hands may rest on your left thigh or touch the wall, whichever is more comfortable. Repeat with the other leg. This stretches the hip flexors, those muscles that work every time you take a step.

5. Stand up straight facing away from the wall. Straighten and extend the right leg in front of you, flexing the foot (heel down, toes up). Your left leg is slightly bent. Lean forward until you feel the stretch in the right hamstring (back of the thigh). Repeat with the left leg.

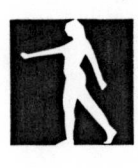 **Instead-of-Cardio Stretch.** The heck with the aerobic workout—you just feel like staying quiet and stretching. That's fine, but warm up the body with some movement first. Cold muscles are difficult to

stretch. You can warm up by marching in place for a couple of minutes, reaching the arms in all directions, or just bustle around the kitchen. Then do the **After-Cardio Stretch** (p. 32) for the lower body, followed by these upper-body exercises:

1. Alternate reaching the arms toward the ceiling slowly, two times each arm.
2. Alternate reaching the arms down your sides slowly, two times each arm.
3. Alternate crossing your arms in front of your chest slowly and opening them as wide as you can, slowly, and repeat.

Easy Does It

Never force a stretch. Go just to your personal limit of comfort. Also never bounce a stretch or do it quickly. Give your muscles time to relax into the stretch. Be especially gentle with yourself first thing in the morning.

Shower Your Back. Don't just sing in the shower: Work your back muscles! Hold a washcloth with both hands at the diagonal corners. Hold one corner steady with your left hand about 6 inches in front of your chest. Pull the other corner back with your right hand toward your rib cage. Pull as hard as you can, squeezing your shoulder blades. Slowly release. Do 8 repetitions, then switch sides.

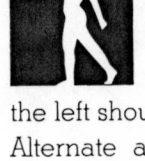 **Shower Your Chest.** After you've worked your back with your washcloth, still holding the corners, cross your wrists and push to the opposite directions (right hand pushing left, left hand pushing right), contracting your pectoral (chest) muscles as if you're trying to make cleavage. Squeeze and release for 8 slow repetitions.

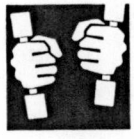 **Neck Roll.** You can do this pleasant stretch in the shower, where the warm water helps to relax stiff muscles, or right after you get out of the shower. Let your head fall gently to the left side until it is close to the left shoulder. Bring it up and let it fall gently to the right side. Alternate a few times. Then slowly roll the head from one shoulder toward the chest and then to the other shoulder. (Do *not* tilt the head back.) Repeat several times.

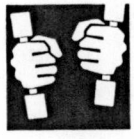 **Shower Scrub.** You might as well clean the shower while you're cleaning yourself. Use a brush to scrub the walls of the shower in a circular motion, working your back and shoulder muscles. Scrub in both directions, and alternate hands.

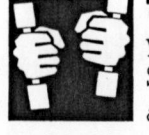 **Towel Your Toes.** While you're toweling off after your morning shower, try this balance exercise: Stand tall on your left leg. With your right leg bent and lifted, wrap your towel around your right foot and pull it up in front of you so it's touching your left thigh. Straighten up and stand tall, abdominals pulled in tight, chest lifted, as you balance on your left leg and dry your right foot, calf, and thigh. Change legs. Balance exercises like this help to strengthen your abdominals and the leg you're standing on.

Shave Your Abs. Isometrically contract your abdominal muscles while you're shaving your face, underarms, or legs (depending on gender and shaving preference!). That means you exhale and pull your abdominal muscles in firmly, as if you are pulling on a pair of jeans that are too tight. Hold your abdominals in, breathing shallowly, for 6 to 10 seconds. Take a deep breath and release the contraction for 4 seconds while you rinse your razor, then contract again and continue shaving. When you're done, lift your chest, lower your shoulders, pull your abs in again—and hold that fine posture all day long. This exercise strengthens your abdominal muscles, improves your posture, and helps you avoid lower-back pain. Time: 10 to 14 seconds per repetition, total 2 to 5 minutes. Caution: If you're not a morning person and you shave with one eye open, protect your jugular vein from that highly sharpened piece of steel by doing the abdominal contractions only when you're rinsing the razor.

================= **Toothbrush Trick** =================

If you keep meaning to go to the health club before work but you never get there, try this gimmick: Keep your comb, toothbrush, and deodorant in your car, buried in your gym bag. You can't get ready for work without them, so you might as well go to the club as you planned.

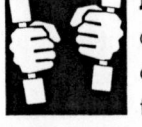 **Beginner's Bun Blow-Dry.** If the idea of balancing on one leg in **Bun Blow-Dry** below takes far too much coordination and concentration, do isometric contractions: Squeeze and release the buttock muscles (4 seconds squeeze, 4 seconds release) with both feet planted solidly on the floor as you dry your hair.

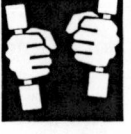 **Bun Blow-Dry.** While you're blow-drying your hair, your arms and shoulders are getting a workout, but the rest of your body is just hanging out doing nothing. You can work your buttocks this way: Stand up straight, abdominals pulled in and buttocks squeezed together. While you hold the hair dryer in your right hand, hold the sink with your left hand, bend your left knee, and lift your left foot off the floor so that it is aiming at the wall directly behind

you. Flex your foot (that is, bend your ankle so that the top of your foot moves toward your lower shin) and press your heel toward the back wall. Keep your buttocks tucked in and forward. Your leg will move just a few inches. Press for 4 seconds, release for 4 seconds, and repeat until your hair is half dry. Change arms and legs and continue until your hair is dry and your buttock muscles are wide awake. (If you don't blow-dry your hair, you can do this while you're doing whatever else you do at the sink.)

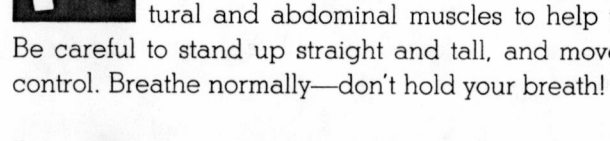 **Advanced Bun Blow-Dry.** Do Bun Blow-Dry (p. 37), but do not hold on to the sink. Tighten your abdominals and lift your chest, using the back postural and abdominal muscles to help you balance. Be careful to stand up straight and tall, and move slowly, with control. Breathe normally—don't hold your breath!

Erotic Exercise. We'd be remiss if we didn't recommend morning sex as a terrific energizer. Here's one exercise you won't be eager to terminate, so you might want to reset the alarm before you get . . . warmed up. Okay, making love doesn't burn many calories, but it's a lovely way to get the blood moving in the morning. Of course if you want to go to sleep after sex, move this exercise to your evening winddown instead of your morning wake-up.

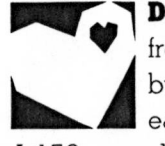 **Dog Walk.** Sure, you can open the door and let Fido frolic on his own. He'll burn plenty of calories; you'll burn none. Or you can let the dog take you for an early morning walk, and you both get your exercise. A 150-pound person who walks the dog for 15 minutes, 5 days a week, will burn 15,750 calories a year—that's a weight loss of 4½ pounds, just from doing that one activity! And if you don't have a dog, walk briskly as if you did. It's not the *dog*, it's the *walk* that burns calories. (You knew that, right?)

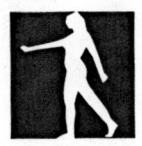 **Stretch As You Dress.** How many muscles can you stretch as you get dressed? Here are some samples, and you'll be able to find others, depending on what you're wearing:

1. Take an extra moment to stretch your chest and shoulders while hooking your bra by pushing your elbows as far back as possible.
2. Before you pull your T-shirt over your head, hold it high in the air.
3. Sit on the bed and pull your bent leg close to you to put on your socks, then extend your leg fully before putting your foot on the floor.
4. Sit on the bed, feet flat on the floor, and bend down to tie your shoes, stretching your back.

12

Chapter 4

9   **Car Stress Busters**   3

6

Y OU'RE STUCK IN THE CAR IN TRAFFIC. Your stress is building. Your time is wasting. Obviously, your main job is driving safely, protecting yourself and fellow motorists, not figuring out how to get a workout. But even when your concentration is on the road, your foot on the pedal, and your hands on the steering wheel, many muscles are just going along for the ride without having to participate. Even with limited motion, that leaves some opportunity for activity. And you'll find you become more alert mentally and physically when you manage to strengthen, release, and stretch a few muscles as you drive (or, even better, stop driving). Rather than feeling cramped, tired, **41** and stressed, your trip can leave you feeling stronger and more rested. Work these exercises into your driving routine when they feel appropriate and safe—but *do not* let your mind or eyes wander from the road!

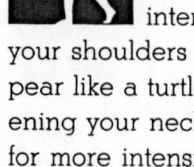 **Shoulder Shrugs.** When our shoulders get tense, they tend to creep up toward our ears, stressing shoulders and neck even more. To counter this, intensify the tension, then release it this way: Hunch your shoulders up toward your ears, making your neck disappear like a turtle's, then push the shoulders way down, lengthening your neck. Brace your hands against the steering wheel for more intensity. Do this 3 times, then leave the shoulders in the "down" position. Your shoulders and neck should feel greatly relieved.

Isometric Contractions Unlimited. How many body parts can you exercise and still drive safely? Try isometric exercises, which means contracting the muscles without taking them through a range of motion. You can tighten your thighs without moving your leg, for example, isometrically contracting the quadriceps (front of the thighs), holding the contraction for a few seconds, then releasing it. Other areas that respond well to isometric contractions in the car are the buttocks, upper arms, shoulders, and abdominals.

Tension Terminator

Most of us have areas we tend to tense when we're driving, such as the neck, jaw, or shoulders. Identify your tension-holding area, and consciously relax it every few minutes. If you can reach it while you're driving, massage the area frequently.

Ab Alert. You can give yourself an abdominal workout and strengthen your postural muscles throughout your drive. Sit up tall, pull your abs in, and lift your chest and rib cage. Ah, perfect posture. As a constant reminder and to make this a habit, adjust your rearview mirror so you can see out of it only in this position. Keep your abs alert by pulling them in and lifting the rib cage as you exhale, then releasing slowly as you inhale.

Arm and Hand Stretch. Do you find you're white-knuckling your commute by gripping the steering wheel? This doesn't get you to your job any faster, but it does tense your hands, wrists, and arms—just what you *don't* want before a day of work, especially if you work at a computer. Reach toward the windshield with one arm (the other arm is continuing to steer), then circle the wrist in both directions. Relax the hand on the steering wheel and open the fingers, then close them into a fist, then open them again. Change arms. Keep your shoulders down and relaxed throughout these exercises.

Car Comfort

Increase your driving comfort and decrease fatigue and stress with these tips from fitness expert and lifestyle coach David Essel, M.S. (*www.davidessel.com*):

- Adjust your neck rest, seat, and steering wheel at the optimum positions for comfort and safety.
- Sit upright; don't slump. Sitting hunched puts stress on the spine and neck and leads to backache and fatigue. Sit tall with your spine, neck, and head aligned and your shoulders back. (Make this a habit when you're standing, too.)
- If your car seat does not permit you to sit up comfortably, roll a towel behind your lower back, or buy a contoured backrest.
- Try the beaded seat covers. These not only feel good, they increase air circulation and let perspiration evaporate instead of sticking you to the seat.
- Invest in high-quality sunglasses to avoid glare and eye fatigue. Get the kind that blocks out both UVA and UVB rays.
- Wear shoes that breathe and allow you to wiggle your toes.
- Wear loose-fitting, nonbinding clothing, preferably beltless. Dressing in layers lets you adjust to temperature changes. If you wear shorts on a hot day, put a towel under your legs to avoid sticking to the seat.
- Wear sun block if you drive with an open window.

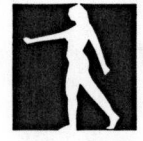 **Flexible Face.** Many of us clench the jaw without realizing it as a reaction to tension, but actually, this only makes stress worse. Stretch your facial muscles by opening up your face with an exaggerated look of surprise—eyes wide, jaw wide, mouth stretched wide open—then release and relax. Do this whenever your commute drives you crazy. Caution: The driver in front of you looking in the rearview mirror will get a startling view of your facial contortions, so either avoid this move in heavy traffic or at least smile like a normal person afterwards. You might also avoid this exercise when a highway patrol person is alongside.

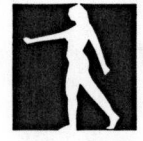 **Get Out and Stretch a Minute.** You've reached your destination (finally!). Take a minute to revitalize with this 60-second stretch as soon as you get out of your car:

- Stretch your arms up toward the sky, alternating high reaches.
- Hold your arms horizontally out to the side and circle them back a few times, then forward.
- Roll your shoulders back and clasp your hands behind you, pulling back until your shoulders release.
- Extend your arms out to the sides again, and twist your upper body very slowly from the waist. (If you have a bad back, however, pivot the feet and turn the whole body instead of twisting at the waist.)

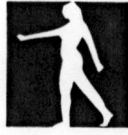 **Red Light Releases.** Stoplights might be aggravating when you're in a hurry, but they're fine opportunities to stretch a few muscles. Put the car in park and try one of these at each light:

- **Neck:** Slowly drop your head to one side toward your shoulder, then straighten up and drop it to the other side. Alternate sides until the light is about to change.
- **Back:** Round your back, then arch it. Alternate arching and rounding.
- **Leg:** Point your foot to stretch your shin, then flex it to stretch your calf. Alternate pointing and flexing. If you have room, straighten out your leg.
- **Feet:** Rotate your ankles. If you have room in your shoes, wiggle your toes.

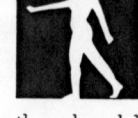 **Shoulder Ripple.** At a stoplight or in a super-slow traffic jam, roll and ripple the shoulders (undulate the shoulders in all directions). Next, hold onto the bottom of the seat with one hand and pull, stretching the shoulders downward. Change arms. Then push both shoulders back by squeezing the shoulder blades toward each other. Relax the shoulders completely for the rest of the trip (or, if you can't, repeat this exercise).

Longer Trips

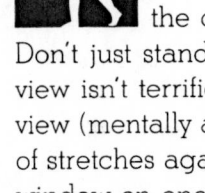**Scenic Stretch.** If you have a drive that lasts more than 1 or 2 hours, plan for a stop to get out and stretch your limbs for a few minutes. Ideally, stop the car at a scenic spot with a breathtaking view. Don't just stand and look—*stretch* and look! But even if the view isn't terrific, the stretch will feel great and improve the view (mentally as well as visually). Do the following 5 minutes of stretches against your car. Before you begin, roll down the window on one car door, and shut the door so you can hold on to the sill. (If you'd like to get as far away from your car as possible, you can do these stretches against a tree.) Hold each stretch for 15 to 30 seconds.

- **Back and Arm Stretch.** Stand an arm's length away from the car door. Lean forward at the waist and hold on to the sill of the open window. Your body should be bent at the hips at about a 90-degree angle. Slightly bend your knees and push your weight away from the car, breathing deeply.
- **Chest and Shoulder Stretch.** Turn around so your back is toward the car door and you're holding on to the sill behind you. Roll your shoulders back and lean your body forward away from the car, chest thrust forward.

- **Calf Stretch.** Face the car and hold the sill with both hands, standing close to the car. Bend the left leg slightly as you step the right leg back as far as it can go with the heel pressed down. You'll feel a stretch in the right calf. Then bring the right leg forward a few inches and slightly bend the right knee, keeping the heel down. You'll feel the stretch go lower in the calf. Repeat both positions with the left leg.

- **Quad Stretch.** Face the car and hold the sill with the left hand. Reach back with the right hand and bend the right knee with the foot behind you until you can hold on to your right ankle (or sock or pant leg, if you can't reach the ankle). Try to keep the thighs together and straighten the back. You'll feel the stretch in the front of the right thigh. Repeat with the left leg.

- **Hip Flexor Stretch.** Face the car and hold the sill with one or both hands. Step back with the right leg. Keeping the left knee bent and directly over the ankle, slide the right leg back until you sink into a lunge, right toes on the ground, right heel lifted. Bend the right knee just to your point of comfort. Don't let the left knee go forward of the foot to avoid stress to the knee. Change legs.

- **Hamstring Stretch.** Stand about 3 to 4 feet behind the car. Put your right heel on the bumper, keeping a very slight bend in the knee. Lean forward until you feel the stretch in the back of the right thigh, your hands resting on your right thigh. Repeat with the left leg.

- **Lower Back Stretch.** Stand close to the car, touching it with your left hand for support. Bring your right knee up toward the chest until you can hook your right arm underneath it. Pull the leg in closer until your lower back stretch says, "Ummmm." Repeat with the left leg. (If this position is awkward, prop your lifted foot against the car and lean forward, rounding your back.)

Mental Fitness

Relaxing your mind without losing your focus is essential for deflecting travel stress and keeping your tension level down. Here are some strategies:

- Leave 10 to 15 minutes early for every hour of expected travel.
- Listen to soothing music to calm you, recorded books to stimulate your mind, or vibrant music to energize you, whichever you need.
- The next time you want to honk the horn at someone, count to 10 slowly first. Then don't honk.
- Face a tension-provoking situation with this philosophy: If you can do something to control it, do so. If it's out of your control, release it. Let it go.
- Breathe! Slow down your breathing to relax. Never hold your breath!

Fit Wheels, Will Travel: A Guide to Healthy Car Trips

Car travel is great for seeing the sights, traveling according to your own schedule, and stopping where and when you want; but sitting in a car for hours is physically uncomfortable and often emotionally stressful. If you finish your vacation day feeling cramped, tense, and aching, what's the point? Your vacation is supposed to revitalize you—not drain your energy and send you home more tired than when you left. By incorporating fitness minutes—and good eating habits—into your trip, you'll return stronger, healthier, and more rested.

Pedal Sightseeing. Put a bike rack on your car and carry bicycles. Each time you pass through an interesting town (without heavy traffic), explore it by bicycle. You'll get plenty of exercise and see sights that you'd miss in the car. You'll also travel longer distances than you can on foot. Be sure to carry a good bicycle lock and water.

Rest Stop Romps. Stop for brisk exercise activity breaks every 1 or 2 hours. Choose a rest stop or scenic spot along the way, or head into town (whatever town you might be passing through) in search of a park, playground, quiet country road—anywhere you can get out of the car and move around vigorously. If you plan your exercise break ahead, you'll have more options: Keep a

Frisbee, jump rope, rubber ball, or basketball in the car, for example. Be sure to wear walking or running shoes. Even 5 minutes of activity will invigorate you mentally as well as physically. After 30 minutes, you'll feel like a new person.

Prepare for Hunger Pangs

Rather than relying on what you'll find at rest stops, plan ahead and carry healthful, low-fat foods. Eating the high-fat, high-salt, high-sugar snacks you usually find on the road will leave you feeling sluggish, bloated, and irritable—and send you home with extra pounds on your belly. Before you leave on your trip, pack some nutritious foods that travel well in a cooler: fresh and dried fruits, cut-up fresh vegetables, frozen bagels. Other nutritious snacks that don't need cooling are dry cereal (great as an out-of-the-box snack), rice cakes, and sunflower seeds. Also carry plenty of water.

Picnic Power

If you're traveling with a companion and especially with children, pack for a picnic along the way—much more fun than visiting a chain restaurant that's just the same as the one you have at home. And a picnic will let the kids run around instead of making them sit in a restaurant after sitting in a car for hours. Instead of leaving a restaurant bored, cranky, and crazy from lack of activity, the kids are likely to be cheerful and maybe even tired enough to sleep in the car.

12

Chapter 5

9 **Work
Workouts** 3

6

PEOPLE WITH SEDENTARY JOBS tend to get groggy, tense, stiff, and less productive as the day wears on. Taking frequent exercise breaks will help you avoid a stiff neck, sore back, and repetitive stress injuries and make the day go faster. It will also make you more productive, because your mental alertness as well as physical energy will improve, and you'll get more high-quality work done. Companies in Japan, for example, realize the bottom-line benefit of employee fitness—many start their workday with mandatory group exercise. Some American companies have state-of-the-art fitness centers and encourage employees to take exercise breaks. Others organize employee sports or provide onsite exercise classes. But even if a structured fitness break is out of the question at your worksite, you can squeeze physical activity into your workday, 1 or 2 minutes here, 5 to 10 minutes there.

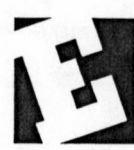 **Walk to Work.** Impossible—you live 1 hour's commute from work, you say? Take public transportation, get off a stop or two from work, and walk the rest of the way. If you drive, park a few blocks from work or at least at the far end of the company parking lot or garage. Alternative: Park your car at the location of a stop you want to make after work—post office, coffee house, bagel shop—rather than at your own workplace. Hoof it to work, then back to your after-work spot. Leave your car where it's easy to find parking, even if—especially if—it's a mile or two away from work. Instead of trying to get as close as possible, try to get as much exercise as possible. You'll feel better, have time to think, and be more productive when you get there. And you'll burn calories and get fitter with every step you take.

Stand and Deliver. As ergonomic as your chair might be, get out of it as often as possible while you work or study. You'll feel less tired and your brain will work better if you take "standing breaks" at least every hour; and, if possible, work standing up for 5 to 10 minutes. You'll burn 25 percent more calories than sitting down. To protect your back, don't lean over your desk. Instead, find tasks that let you stand upright, like returning phone calls, reading reports, or jotting notes using a clipboard.

Stair Climb. Don't call it a flight of stairs—it's a foot-operated cardio machine! A 150-pound person burns 17½ calories per minute walking up stairs. So skip the elevator and climb your way to your office. If you work on the top floor of a high-rise, take the elevator most of the way, then walk as many of those flights as you can manage.

Pencil Toss. If coworkers are whispering at the water cooler about your workout antics, here's a subtle approach to getting a back stretch. Turn your chair away from your desk so you have room in front of you. "Accidentally" drop your pencil on the floor. Lower your chest over your thighs and reach for your pencil. If you need more stretch, flick the pencil farther away and keep reaching. Take your time picking it up, exhaling into the stretch. If no one's watching—or if you don't care if they are—stay in the stretch for 10 to 30 seconds, relaxing and sinking into the stretch each time you exhale. This exercise stretches the lower back and middle back.

Pace Your Work. Which work tasks can you do pacing instead of sitting? If you can pace while you work—while talking on the phone, brainstorming, or discussing projects with colleagues or clients, for example—you'll burn almost four times as many calories as you will sitting.

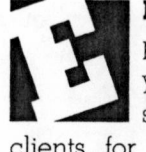

Speaker Phone Push-Ups. If your work involves frequent phone calls, here's a way to improve your upper-body strength and make productive use of time otherwise wasted. Each time you make a phone call, turn on the speaker phone after you dial. Do push-ups against the desk while you wait for the person to answer. Place your hands about shoulder-width apart on the desk. Walk your feet away until your body makes a diagonal line from desk to floor. Keeping your back neutral (that is, not rounded or arched), your abdominals tight, your chest high, and your shoulders down, bend your elbows, lowering your chest toward the desk. Exhale, straightening your elbows (do not lock them) and pushing yourself away from the desk. Repeat until the person answers. (Careful of the heavy breathing when you introduce yourself!)

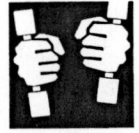 **Advanced Phone Push-Ups.** You don't have to have a speaker phone to do **Speaker Phone Push-Ups** (p. 56). Do one-armed push-ups. Change arms with each call. This exercise strengthens the chest, arms, and shoulders and amazes your coworkers.

Hand Delivery. Instead of sending an e-mail to a coworker 1 minute away, get up and deliver your message personally. Taking 4 minutes to compose and send an e-mail burns only 2 to 3 calories. Walking for 1 minute, then standing up talking to your colleague for 3 minutes, burns 6 calories. It all adds up. Plus you'll get the kinks out of your back.

Walk a Colleague. Instead of sitting in a meeting with a coworker or client, have your discussion while you take a walk together—outside if you can, but even in the hallway if necessary. Your mind will work better, and you'll get a little fitness break.

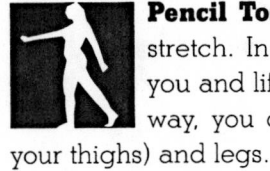 **Pencil Toss with Legs.** Do the **Pencil Toss** (p. 55) stretch. In addition, straighten your legs in front of you and lift your toes while you relax your back. This way, you can also stretch the hamstrings (backs of your thighs) and legs.

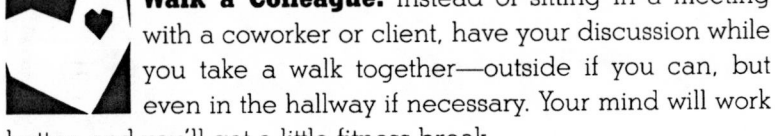

Work Workouts

Burn 'Em, Don't Eat 'Em. It's time for your mid-morning break, and your energy level is low. You reach for coffee and doughnuts to give yourself a little rush. But doing so—if you react to the combination of caffeine, sugar, flour, and fat in these foods the way most of us do—will ensure that your energy level will take a dive again in a couple of hours. A better plan is to just say no to the pastries and caffeine, change to comfortable shoes, and push your tired body out your office door at break time. If you can get outside, walk around the block as briskly as possible. If not, do the same thing in a conveniently located corridor. You'll energize physically and mentally, and do better work when you get back to your chair. At a pace of 4 miles per hour, a 150-pound person can burn 85 calories in 15 minutes. And you'll avoid the calories and fat you would have eaten.

Your Own Step Class. Whether you have a 10-minute break or only 30 seconds to exercise, change into a pair of comfortable, rubber-soled shoes (you keep those at the ready in your office, don't you?), and get to the nearest flight of stairs. Walk up a flight or two, walk down a flight or two—or more. Be careful to keep your posture upright and hold your abdominals tight; don't slouch or lean into the next step.

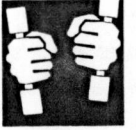 **Floor Pickup.** Oops, you "accidentally" dropped a report on the floor. Squat down and up several times before picking it up. To avoid knee stress, keep your derrière way back and don't let your knees go forward of the toes. For even less stress on the knees, use a wide-legged stance.

Calories Not Eaten

If you grab an exercise break instead of a pastry, give yourself credit for the calories you're not eating as well as those you're burning. According to the Center for Science in the Public Interest, Cinnabon's cinnamon roll, for example, has 670 calories and 34 grams of fat, equivalent to eating a Big Mac and a hot fudge sundae. Au Bon Pain's pecan roll has 800 calories and 45 grams of fat, as much as Denny's Grand Slam breakfast (2 slices bacon, 2 sausage links, 2 eggs, 2 pancakes). Starbucks' cinnamon scone has 530 calories and 26 grams of fat—the equivalent of two pork chops and mashed potatoes with butter. If you don't eat your usual snack that has, say, 700 calories, you'll lose a pound a week just from that omission! And if you add walking instead of eating, you'll lose even more.

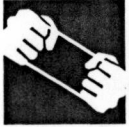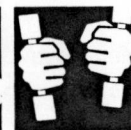 **Pump Rubber.** Keep Dyna-Bands—latex strips of different intensities created expressly for strength training and stretching—or other resistance bands at

work. Doing a strength exercise with these bands will pep you up better than caffeine. Do 1 minute each of the following exercises:

- **Squat with Bands.** Stand with your heels anchoring down the ends of two bands, holding the other ends at your waist. Bend so that you can hoist the ends up over your shoulders. Your hands hold the ends of the bands in front of your shoulders, while the band goes over and behind your shoulders, down your sides, and to your feet. Shift your weight back as if you were about to sit in a chair. Squat down, keeping your back neutral, your chest up, and your weight over your heels. Don't let your knees come forward of your toes. Squeeze your buttock muscles as you straighten up. Repeat. This works your thighs and buttocks.
- **Upright Row with Bands.** Stand with your heels anchoring down the ends of two bands. Overlap the free ends of the bands so that you create a flexible barbell under your hands. Pull the overlapped section up toward your chest, keeping your shoulders down. Squeeze your shoulder blades, then slowly release. Repeat. You'll feel the work in your upper back muscles, an area that is frequently over-stretched and underworked during desk work.
- **Seated Row with Bands.** Sit in a chair, the middle of one band anchored under your feet, knees apart, hands holding the ends of the band. Cross the band and exchange hands

so that you're holding opposite ends and the band makes an "X" between your knees. Pull your elbows back until your hands come to your ribs, and squeeze your shoulder blades. Release slowly. Repeat. Keep your back straight and shoulders down throughout the exercise. This works the large muscles of the back. (Learn more about Dyna-Bands and where to order them in the Resources Appendix.)

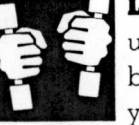 **Skip a Step, Advanced.** In case you don't have enough flights of stairs in your building to challenge you, pump up the intensity by taking the stairs two at a time. This strengthens your thighs and buttocks as well as burning calories at an aerobic pace. Do this on the way up only!

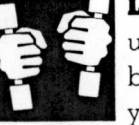 **Lunge the Stairs, Advanced.** Do lunges up (never down!) a flight of stairs. Start by standing on one step, then placing your right foot two steps higher, both legs bent. Push up, straightening both legs and shifting all your weight to your right leg, then place your left foot two steps above your right, bending both legs again. Keep going until you've reached your destination or your legs and buttocks are screaming for mercy. Squeeze your buttocks each time you

straighten up. This strengthens your cardiovascular system, thighs, and buttocks and burns calories briskly. You'll feel energized and your face will have a healthy glow.

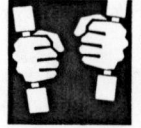 **Grin and Bear It.** Get your exercise while you're working by offering to lift and/or carry anything that needs moving. Change the water jug at the cooler. Move in the new printer and carry out the old. Fetch cartons of supplies for your officemates. Greet the package-delivery service at the door and carry the packages to the proper desks. Your coworkers will think you're Ms. or Mr. Helpful, and you'll get plenty of extra minutes of energizing exercise. Lifting and carrying items strengthens your back, abdominals, arms, and thighs.

Lifting Right

Whether you're lifting dumbbells, a printer, a box of office supplies, or a set of car keys, follow these guidelines to keep your back healthy and safe:

- Keep your back neutral, neither arched nor rounded.
- Lift with your thighs, not your back. Squat down, legs wide, to pick up the object. Pull it in close to you before you straighten up.
- Do not twist and lift at the same time. Face the object before you start to pick it up. Turn your whole body toward the object's destination before you put it down.
- If the object is too heavy to lift safely, get help.

 **Obliques Online.** Use those annoying down times when you're waiting for a file to print or a Web page to load, and work your obliques—the side abdominal muscles that help to shape your waist—at your desk. Lift one knee as you lower the opposite shoulder, exhaling and contracting the obliques. Alternate until duty calls.

Upper-Back Bliss. This upper-back stretch looks odd, but it effectively releases tension between your shoulder blades. Extend your arms in front of your chest, palms facing each other. Cross your wrists—now the backs of your hands are touching. Rotate your wrists until your palms face each other (your elbows will flare out). Lower your shoulders and press your palms together. Slightly round your back to intensify the stretch.

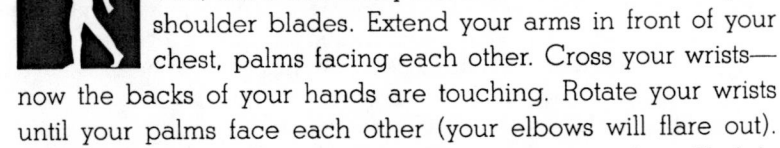 **Junk-Mail Crumple.** Each time you get a piece of junk mail, don't just toss it—crumple it first. Open the envelope and pull out the letter (don't worry—you don't have to read it). Hold it with one hand. Start at one corner and crumple it into your palm, bit by bit, until it's one tight ball. Squeeze it a few times, then drop it in the recycling container. Grab another item with your other hand, and repeat. This strengthens your forearm, relieves wrist tension from overuse at the keyboard, and gives your junk mail some purpose during its very brief time in your life.

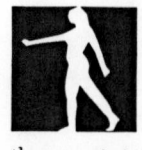 **Ankle Line Dance.** You're on the phone and busily taking notes. Reduce stress and increase circulation with some fancy footwork. Alternate pointing your toes and flexing your feet (toes toward your shins); then rotate your ankles in one direction, then the other. You'll enjoy this even more if you can shed your shoes first.

Keyboard Comfort

If you spend both your workday and your leisure time on the computer, you could develop carpal tunnel syndrome, a common repetitive stress injury resulting from inflammation of the tendons in the wrist and pinching of the median nerve. Symptoms range from burning, tingling, and numbness in the fingers, especially the thumb and the index and middle fingers, to difficulty gripping or making a fist.

Your best bet for avoiding carpal tunnel syndrome is to change your work habits so that you don't stress the wrist. According to the Ergonomics Program at the University of California, San Francisco and Berkeley, the following should help:

- Support your forearms comfortably on the arms of your chair while typing.
- Grasp the mouse lightly and loosely, keeping your wrists straight.
- Keep your elbows near your body and your forearms approximately parallel to the floor, resting on armrests or forearm supports.
- Make sure the slope of the keyboard keeps your wrists straight while you type.
- Type with your hands and wrists hovering lightly above the keyboard.

- Use a wrist pad only to rest your wrists when you're not typing.
- Move your whole arm to press hard-to-reach keys instead of twisting your wrists sideways.
- Press the keys gently, keeping your shoulders, arms, hands, and fingers relaxed.
- Vary your position and tasks frequently. Take breaks every 20 to 30 minutes.

Calf Relief. If you wear high-heeled shoes at work, your calves are contracted whenever you stand or walk. A few times a day, take off your shoes, massage your calves, then stand up and do this stretch: Bend the left leg slightly and step the right foot back as far as it can go with the heel pressed into the floor, keeping the right leg straight. Lean forward slightly until you feel a strong, pleasurable stretch in the right calf. Hold until all tension releases. Then bend the right leg slightly, taking the stretch into the lower calf muscles. When the right calf feels wonderful, switch sides.

Park Your Lunch. Make your lunchtime a real pep-me-up by packing lunch and walking to the closest park. Stride, don't meander. At the park, use the exercise stations or continue walking. Take a break to eat the lunch you brought, then walk back. If the park isn't close enough to fit all this in, you can drive to the park, as long as you walk once you get there. (See Chapter 8 for many more ideas.)

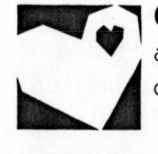

Copy Machine Back Stretch. Making photocopies doesn't have to be wasted time. Face the copy machine and place your hands on top, then walk your feet back (away from the machine), hinging from the hips as you bend forward. Alternate arching and rounding your back.

Carry-Out Workout. Order food by phone for you and your work buddies, and offer to go pick up the chow. See how quickly you can walk there and back.

Desk Quad Stretch. When you get back to your desk after a walking or stair-climbing break, stretch your quadriceps (front of the thighs). Stand up straight and, keeping your thighs together, bend the right knee and hold your right foot (or pant leg, if you can't reach your foot) behind you with your right hand. You're standing on your left foot. Place one hand on the desk for balance if you feel wobbly, but keep standing up straight. After your right thigh feels pleasantly stretched, switch legs.

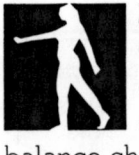 **Balancing Quad Stretch, Advanced.** Do the Desk Quad Stretch (p. 66), but without holding on to the desk. Instead, reach your free hand toward the ceiling, lifting through the abdominals. By adding a balance challenge, you strengthen the postural muscles in the abdominals and back while you're stretching your quadriceps.

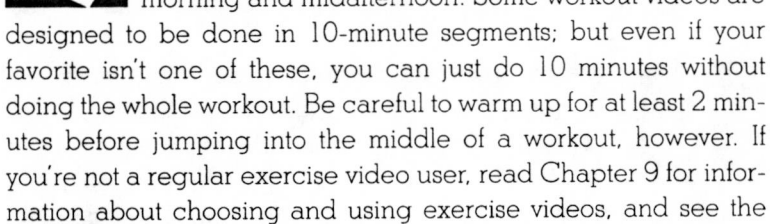 **Home Business Video Blast.** If you work in a home office, keep an exercise videotape cued and ready to go for exercise breaks during the day, especially mid-morning and midafternoon. Some workout videos are designed to be done in 10-minute segments; but even if your favorite isn't one of these, you can just do 10 minutes without doing the whole workout. Be careful to warm up for at least 2 minutes before jumping into the middle of a workout, however. If you're not a regular exercise video user, read Chapter 9 for information about choosing and using exercise videos, and see the Resources Appendix for suggestions about where to order them.

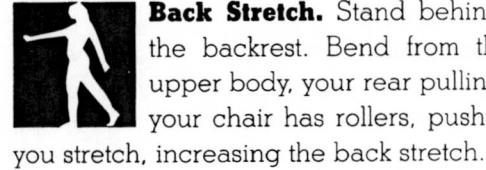 **Back Stretch.** Stand behind your chair, hands on the backrest. Bend from the hips, lowering your upper body, your rear pulling away from the chair. If your chair has rollers, push it a little bit forward as you stretch, increasing the back stretch.

Worksite Wellness

Have you checked into whether your company offers a health promotion program? Many companies, understanding the value of having fit employees, offer incentives for getting in shape, such as partial payment for gym memberships. Ask your human resources department.

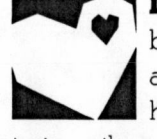 **Lunch Aerobics.** Organize a lunchtime walking or basketball group. You'll not only get your exercise, but also promote camaraderie among your coworkers and have more fun than you'd find in the company cafeteria or the restaurant next door. Sponge off at the sink afterwards.

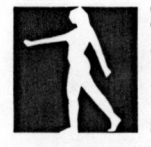 **Hamstring Stretch.** If you've been climbing stairs, this stretch for the hamstrings (back of the thighs) will feel terrific. Stand on your left leg, your right leg straight with your foot on a chair in front of you. Bend and straighten the left leg slowly, increasing and decreasing the stretch in the right hamstring muscles. Then switch legs. Warning: Don't do this on a chair with rollers!

 **Swim and Sandwich.** Head for your community pool and swim laps, take an aqua aerobics class, or do your own pool exercises for 30 minutes at lunch hour. Eat your sandwich on the way back. Even a slow crawl burns 300 calories in a half hour, and it's relaxing.

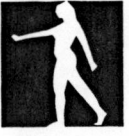 **Chest and Shoulder Stretch.** A problem with desk work is that almost all your work is done in front of you, using the chest and shoulder muscles, usually without stretching them. Sitting in your chair, reach both arms back as far as you can, arching your back. If your backrest is designed to permit this, clasp your hands behind the chair to intensify the stretch. Doing this stretch several times during the day will release tension and make you feel better. It takes no extra time, because you can continue to read the computer monitor or printed report while you stretch.

Mobile Locker Room. Keep a gym bag in your car packed with any clothing or gear you need for your favorite spontaneous sport: basketball, tennis racket, skates, walking/running shoes, sweats, swimsuit, towel, Frisbee, you name it. Instead of driving straight home after work, stop for a fitness fix.

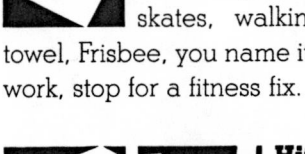 **Hit the Health Club.** You may think that a whirlwind visit to a health club at lunch or after work is worse than no visit at all, but you're dead wrong. Even if you only have time to work out for 15 minutes, that's 75 more minutes of exercise each week than you're getting now. And you'll feel much more clear-headed and energetic in the afternoon.

12

Chapter 6

9   **Getting It**   3
      Together:
      Getting and
      Staying Motivated

6

I T'S EASY TO START AN EXERCISE PROGRAM—many of us have done
it dozens of times! The problem is becoming consistent and
sticking with it. Motivation isn't something you can order
from eBay—you have to find it within yourself and help it grow.
Whether you're motivating yourself to take a walk during
lunchtime, to "just say no" to chocolate after midnight, or to put
some of your hard-earned salary into retirement savings, the
process is similar. You've got to be ready to change, believe in
the value of that change, and commit to doing what it takes to
get there.   **71**

Fortunately, physical activity has many immediate benefits—you feel better, look better, have more energy, and improve your mood, for example. It's easier to stick to an activity program that makes you feel good right away than it is to try to make some other change that leaves you feeling deprived. Still, as pleasurable as it is to be an active person, most of us need help with motivation. Use what works for you here, and you'll be able to lift yourself over the hump when your motivation threatens to wither.

Which Stage of Change?

It's easy to fall into a program because others (spouse, doctor, best friend) have told you that you should. But when you personally are not really ready to make a change, it usually backfires. Be certain that making a change is your idea and that you're ready. It helps to see where you fit in the stages of change that researchers have identified:

1. Precontemplation: You're not seriously considering changing. You're not even thinking about it.
2. Contemplation: You're thinking seriously about making a change, but you're not doing anything about it. Many people stay in this stage for a long time because they cannot imagine themselves behaving differently, or they do not know how to change.
3. Preparation: You've made a choice to take action and you've even started doing it now and then, though not consistently.
4. Action: Yes, you're doing it consistently now! You're walking your talk, taking action.
5. Maintenance: You've been putting your change into action for 6 months or more, which means it has become a habit.

Focus on Internal Motivation

If your motivation originates externally—you're doing it for your spouse or children or employer—it usually leads to guilt, frustration, anger, and often quitting. When you can say honestly, "I'm doing this because I want to—it will make me feel good," then your motivation is internal. If your doctor is telling you to exercise, look for your internal motivation: Why do *you* want to do this? You don't have to be totally convinced—ambivalence is natural. But can you list the personal rewards that make the change worth making? If you can't, you're not ready to change.

Commit to Your Change

Think about what you want to change and how you can make that change in a way that is realistic, meaningful, and enjoyable for you. Make a commitment to your change. Write down your plan for change. Tell family, friends, and maybe coworkers about it because "going public" often makes the commitment feel more real. And they might want to join you in some of your activities.

Affirm Your Change

Write down a personally meaningful affirmation that puts your change into present tense, such as "I am a strong, physically active person who finds joy in movement," or "I exercise many

73

times a day, look forward to it, and feel great afterwards." Picture yourself as the vital, lean, energetic person you are becoming. Post your affirmation where you'll see it often. Memorize it and say it to yourself several times a day.

Set Goals That Are Specific, Realistic, and Attainable

Too often people set goals that end up biting them in the leg. Make sure your goals pass all three of these tests:

- **They're specific.** "I'll start exercising tomorrow" isn't specific. What will you do? "I'll walk for 10 minutes tomorrow and do three of the exercises in Chapter 5, is specific. See the difference? Avoid using the words "try" or "may" or "maybe" in your goals. A specific goal states exactly what you'll do, and you can track afterwards whether or not you did what you promised.
- **They're realistic.** If you're a nonexerciser now, a goal of walking for 30 minutes a day is probably unrealistic. It's just too much for your fitness level now (although you'll be able to do it before long, we promise) and likely will leave you feeling discouraged and ready to exchange your walking shoes for your bedroom slippers. Instead, figure out what you could *successfully* accomplish at your present fitness level and with your schedule—maybe a 15-minute walk plus, later in the day, 5

minutes of 1-minute exercises from this book. Assess not only what you're willing to do, but also what you *can* do.

- **They're attainable.** Make sure your goals are based on action, not wishes. For example, "I will accumulate 30 minutes of exercise over the course of the day using the activities I flagged in this book" is based on action—you are fully in charge of whether or not you achieve your goal. "I will lose 15 pounds this month" is not attainable. It's too high a number for one, but even if it weren't, the rate at which you lose weight is influenced by many factors—genetics, calorie balance, dieting history, fitness level, intensity of exercise, time of month (for women), and others. You just can't control how fast you lose weight. You *can* control how much you exercise and what you eat. Yes, that will result in weight loss eventually, but the point is that your *goal* should be one you're fully in charge of achieving, exactly as you stated it. Break your big goals into smaller, manageable action steps—small steps lead to lasting changes.

Know Why

Look behind your goals to the reasons why they're important. What do you want to accomplish long-term and why? If you want to lose weight, what will that change in your life? Do you want to be healthier? Have more clothing styles to choose from? Look more youthful and attractive? Have a more active social life? Have more energy? If you want to be stronger, what will that do for you? Stop you from fatiguing so fast? Let you play with your grandchildren more actively? Keep you independent late in life? Understanding the reasons behind your goals will help you stay on track.

Write It Down

Writing down your goals and action steps makes them happen, says Tina B. Tessina, Ph.D., psychotherapist and author of *The REAL 13th Step* (Rev. edition, Career Press, 2001) and many other books. Here's why:

When you visualize and write down exactly and clearly what you want to accomplish, you direct your brain to pay attention. You actually program your brain to focus on your goals.

To make it easy to include exercise in your life, suggests Tessina, write down your goal—such as "I will walk an extra 15 minutes a day"—and picture yourself walking and enjoying it. Perhaps you picture parking a few blocks away from work and walking the rest of the way, or getting off the bus or subway one stop early, or walking to a restaurant or art museum for lunch, or taking a sandwich to a nearby park, or walking the dog a bit longer than usual after work. If you picture yourself walking and enjoying it, you'll soon find that you're noticing more ways you can add in walking without stressing about it.

Plan for Success

Prepare for your exercise activities. If you're planning to walk at work, be sure you have comfortable clothes and walking shoes with you. If you plan to work out with a video in the morning, clear the living room the night before. If you plan to exercise when you get home from work, don't settle down to watch the news and eat a snack first. Alert anyone else who might distract you with other responsibilities that you have an important appointment.

Buddy Up

Many people make progress more easily if they have a support system. Can you identify one or two friends, colleagues, or relatives who have similar goals? If so, get together and help each other achieve your goals. Ideally, you can exercise together—it's much easier to "show up" when someone is counting on you. But even if your support system is a long-distance phone call or an Internet buddy, you can motivate each other, share goals, plan together, and check up on how the other is doing.

Make It a Habit

Believe it or not, if you're careful to be consistent while it feels foreign, you'll discover that exercise will become a habit. It will not be an effort any longer—in fact, it will feel more natural to be physically active than to be sedentary. But until you get to that point, you'll need to use all the tricks you can muster to stick to it for the first 6 months and create consistency so your body and your mind will learn to expect physical activity and look forward to it.

Weight Loss Truths

If you're aiming for weight loss, keep this truth in mind: A 3,500-calorie deficit equals 1 pound of weight loss. That means that if you use up 3,500 calories more than you consume, you'll lose a pound. If your goal is a pound a week, which is realistic with some effort, you can accomplish that in these ways:

- Eat 500 fewer calories per day.
- Increase your physical activity by 500 calories per day.
- Eat 250 fewer calories per day plus increase your physical activity by 250 calories per day.

If you're content to lose weight more slowly and you'd rather not change your eating habits, you can still lose weight, though not as quickly, by making your daily life more active. By including an extra half hour of moderate physical activity most days of the week, you're burning about 1,000 extra calories—that's the loss of a pound in about 3½ weeks. It might not seem fast, but realize that you'll lose about 15 pounds a year this way! Now, that's motivating!

Be careful not to use your newfound exercise habit as an excuse to eat more. A large order of French fries is 400 calories—an easy way to sabotage your good intentions and put the weight back on. After all, it takes 90 minutes of walking at 3 miles per hour to burn off those French fries, which took just a few minutes to eat. Weigh the consequences in your mind before eating high-calorie foods, so you don't have to weigh them as you stand on the scale.

Anticipate Obstacles

What are the likely roadblocks you'll encounter as you put your plan into action? Consider not only external roadblocks (work schedule, family responsibilities, weather, a bike tune-up, and so on), but also internal barriers—your personal feelings and attitudes that could get in your way. For example, you might feel guilty or selfish taking time for yourself, or you might doubt that you'll stick to this program. Write down all such obstacles you're likely to encounter.

Prepare for Overcoming Obstacles

For each obstacle on your list, figure out a plan for not letting it derail your program. If your spouse and children worry that you will be taking time away from them, for example, take time to discuss your program with them, explaining why it's important to you. Figure out ways to involve them, like family hikes or bike rides on the weekend. If you can't see your way to overcoming a particular obstacle, talk to a trusted friend, family member, or counselor about it, or rethink how you can accomplish your goal in a slightly different way.

Don't Punish Yourself for Lapses

This isn't going to work perfectly. You're human. If you fall off the exercise wagon, climb back on without beating yourself up.

You're not deficient in character, willpower, or fortitude. Lapses are part of the process. Each one is an opportunity to learn what sends you off track so you can avoid it next time. Learn to say, "So what? Today I'll do better," if you missed a day or didn't do what you resolved. But, of course, don't let one lapse become a string of lapses—get right back on track. What counts is what you do 80 percent of the time. And if the day runs away from you, remember even if it seems like a drop in the bucket, doing *something* is better than doing nothing.

Log Your Minutes

You might find it helpful to log your exercise sessions in a datebook or journal you reserve for this purpose or to make a weekly chart that includes date, type of exercise/activity, total minutes, and how you felt during and after the activity. Try this if you'll get a feeling of accomplishment from seeing how you accumulate exercise minutes.

Track Your Progress

If you have trouble sticking to a program because your goals seem so far away, select a program that gives you immediate feedback. For example, strength training lets you see impressive improvements within the first few weeks, especially if you record the difficulty and number of repetitions you are able to do. You can also chart your speed on the rowing machine, your miles walking, or your minutes on the exercise bike. Even just keeping an exercise log or marking exercise sessions on your calendar will often keep you on track. If you're trying to lose weight, track your progress with a tape measure or by clothing fit rather than relying on the scale. Choose an item of clothing that fits tightly now, and then try it on every two weeks.

Avoiding Holiday Hijack

Most people average 7 pounds of weight gain from Thanksgiving to New Year's Day. Every New Year's Day, millions of people stare at the mirror and ask themselves with a groan, "What have I done?" This doesn't have to happen to you! Instead of sinking your shape-up program over the holidays, keep it afloat with these strategies.

- **Stress Attack? Cardio Defense!** Aerobic exercise will reduce stress, increase circulation, and release endorphins—"feel good" chemicals in the brain. Your world will be brighter—and so will you. Get your heart rate up with brisk walking, bicycling, dancing, skating, stair climbing, hiking, or playing your favorite sport.
- **Reach for a Stroll, not a Roll!** Instead of seconds of food, take minutes on foot! Leave your plate, and go for a 10- to 20-minute walk. By the time you return, your appetite will be under control. Hint for restaurant eating: Park a 10-minute walk away. You'll arrive less eager to overeat, and you'll have to walk off part of your dessert to get back to your car.

- **No Time to Exercise? Take Two!** If you can't fit your usual selection of exercises into your day, don't beat yourself up. Just do 2 minutes here, 2 minutes there. You're just trying to maintain, not make great fitness progress.
- **Move Before Eating.** Physical activity right before eating will make you want to eat less—and the calories you eat will be burned faster.
- **Vigorous Visitors.** Don't let your best intentions die when you have guests from out of town. Show them the sights of your town—on foot. Walk them around your local park. Take them to your line-dance class. Without being heavy-handed about it, try to incorporate physical activity into the things you do together.
- **Give Gifts That Fit, Not Fatten.** Help a loved one get or stay in shape with a gift that suits an active lifestyle, not one that sabotages it. Forget the fruitcake and cookies, and give a healthful gift: a motivating fitness book (like this one!), exercise video, or heart-healthy recipe book; exercise accessories like weight gloves, walking shoes, or a bicycle rearview mirror; a session with a personal trainer; a personal "gift certificate" for a hike, bike ride, or evening out dancing with you. Use your imagination!
- **Get Back to Basics.** As soon as the holidays are over, return immediately to your usual routine of physical activity. Don't let it go an extra day, which can turn into an extra week, an extra month, and so on. If you do get behind, though, don't use that as an excuse to abandon your program. Just start again.

Reward Yourself

Give yourself credit not only for goals reached, but also for just sticking with it. Drop a dollar or a quarter into a jar each time you exercise. Double it if you didn't feel like exercising but did it anyway. Then when your loot fills the jar, reward yourself with something that will make exercising easier or more fun: new athletic shoes, motivating music, dance lessons, comfortable walking shorts . . . you get the idea.

Take Credit

If you get discouraged and are tempted to quit, think back to your first week getting active: You felt weak and clumsy. You thought you'd never have the stamina to do your errands on foot. The Dyna-Bands snapped in your face because you couldn't get the hang of how to stand on the ends. Stretching felt like an Olympic event. Give yourself credit for what you've accomplished already and for overcoming the biggest obstacle: getting started. Surely you don't want to lose the ground you've gained. It's much easier to keep going than to start all over again. But the good news is that even if you do have to start all over again, your body will remember what being active feels like, will want to get there again, and will respond much more quickly the second time than the first time.

Help a Friend

One way to see your progress in a new way and rediscover the joy of exercise is to help someone else get on the path to fitness.

Take an inactive friend along on your next walk or share an easy activity with a sedentary coworker. Taking a newcomer under your wing and sharing the joy of movement might be enough to help you discover it anew.

Beat the 6-Month Barrier

Half of all people who join an exercise program drop out in the first 6 months—and half of those drop out before the first session. (They join a gym but never go, or they buy a jogging suit but wear it only for lounging around the house, for example.) If you break the 6-month barrier, however, you're likely to make exercise a lifelong habit. Even if you drop out at some point, you're likely to resume your program later. So make that 6-month commitment today!

12

Chapter 7

9   Errand   3
Energizers

6

GETTING AROUND TOWN can be a perfect opportunity to accumulate exercise minutes if you look at errands as an opportunity to be active. Spark up your shopping, banking, and other necessary outings with extra spurts of physical activity that take just a few seconds to a few minutes each. All of these contribute toward making you an active person with energy to burn (literally!), a lively step, a healthy body, and a clear mind.

Park and Walk. Visiting a mall or shopping center? Don't troll for the parking spot closest to the store where you're intending to shop. Instead, park in a space way at the far end of the parking lot or garage. Not only will you get more exercise getting to the store and back, but since most people like to park close, you'll have an easier time finding a spot and less chance of your car getting dinged by an impatient or careless driver.

Curb Your Calves. Anytime you're walking and have to wait for a street light, do extra-slow calf raises on a curb, your heels hanging off the edge: Push up slowly onto your toes, and slowly release back down—4 seconds up and 4 seconds down. Tighten your abs and buttocks to help you balance so you don't have to grab a signpost.

Drive Not Thru. Give up drive-through windows. Park the car and walk into the bank, burning almost five times more calories than you do sitting in your car. Even better, park in some other bank's parking lot and walk to yours. You don't have to racewalk—even a leisurely stroll at 2 miles per hour burns more than twice as many calories as sitting in your car. Of course, faster walking burns even more.

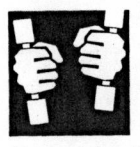

Tight Abs. Do isometric abdominal intervals any-time, anywhere you stand or sit. Contract your abs six times slowly (6-second repetition), then six times quickly (2-second rep), then six times super-slowly (10-second rep), and repeat.

Shop Till You Drop. Park your car at your last errand, not your first, so you won't be tempted to drive from one spot to the next. Ask for shopping bags with handles for easy carrying, or bring your own mesh or canvas shopping bags. If you're halfway through your errands and already carrying plenty of packages, make a detour to your car, park the parcels, then jog to the next errand on your list. The more you walk, the more calories you burn (especially if you're carrying packages) and the more energized you feel.

Subtle Butt. Isometrically contract your gluteals—squeeze your rear end muscles—any time you're stuck waiting: in the post office line, at the dentist's office, wherever. You can do these sitting or standing, but if you're standing and wearing tight jeans and the person behind you winks or grins, you may be attracting more attention than you think. (Check this out in a full-length mirror at home before you take it on the road—it's not as subtle as it feels!)

Errand Energizers

87

Hoof, Don't Surf. Shopping online is convenient, but if you walk from shop to shop in the mall or canvas your favorite warehouse store for 1 hour, you'll burn 145 to 240 calories, depending on speed and how frequently you stop to window-shop or finger the merchandise—as opposed to 30 calories for clicking your way through the Web.

Errand Excess

Our recommendations in this chapter boil down to one easy-to-follow theme: *Do what you'd do anyway, but more actively.*

Instead of choosing the easiest, most energy-conserving way to perform an action, figure out how you can do it expending the most calories. Stand instead of sit. Walk instead of stand. Carry what you can instead of rolling it in a cart. Make your muscles work, even when you could get away with ignoring them. Make extra trips. Burn more calories. Do more than you have to.

Yes, this method will make your errands take a little longer than if you park close to the store, run in, run out, and accomplish every task as efficiently as possible with minimal muscle power. But at what cost? You will save a few minutes and expend very few calories, getting no long-term health benefits or short-term energy benefits. With our "do it more actively" method, you might get your whole 30-minute, daily allotment of exercise just running your errands; and you'll finish up more energized and less stressed than when you started. And you surely will enjoy your errands more!

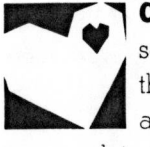 **Case the Joint.** Instead of starting your shopping as soon as you arrive at a mall or shopping center, take the first 10 to 15 minutes to walk briskly all the way around the shopping area as fast as possible. You can peek in the windows as you breeze by, but don't stop. Then return afterwards to the stores that caught your interest. Likewise, when you first enter a large store like a grocery store or warehouse store, speedwalk the perimeter before you start shopping.

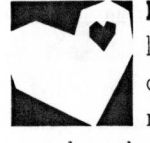 **Loads of Laundry.** Whether you're using the laundry machines in the basement of your apartment or at the public Laundromat, make several trips from your apartment or from your car so that your feet get extra mileage from this chore.

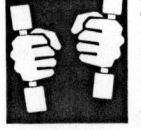 **Don't Just Stand There.** When you take the escalator, don't just go along for the ride. Walk up or down as if it were a regular staircase. You'll burn more than seven times as many calories as just standing there. Escalator etiquette: Pass on the left.

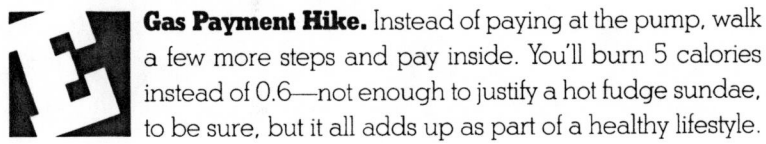 **Gas Payment Hike.** Instead of paying at the pump, walk a few more steps and pay inside. You'll burn 5 calories instead of 0.6—not enough to justify a hot fudge sundae, to be sure, but it all adds up as part of a healthy lifestyle.

Errand Energizers

89

Lose the Lift. Taking the stairs instead of the elevator is just as useful for errands as it is at work (see Chapter 5). Whether you're visiting the doctor, dentist, or therapist, skip the elevator and walk the flights to your appointment. Climbing stairs burns almost ten times more calories than riding the elevator and two to three times as many calories as walking on flat ground. Climbing stairs is as intense an activity as jogging or playing racquetball. And it will shape up your legs!

Subway Shuffle, Bus Boogie. If you're taking public transportation, leave the seats for people who really need them. Stand during your ride, concentrating on strengthening your abs, back, and thighs by stabilizing your body during stops, curves, and lurches. To do this, tighten and lift your abdominal muscles, lift your chest, lengthen your back, and tighten your buttocks and thighs. Focus your gaze on something immobile—a banner ad or some interesting graffiti—rather than something moving, like another passenger or the sights out the window. You'll need to hold onto the pole or strap so that you're not thrown into the lap of another rider, but work toward getting enough core (torso) strength and balance awareness to barely hold on rather than using a death grip.

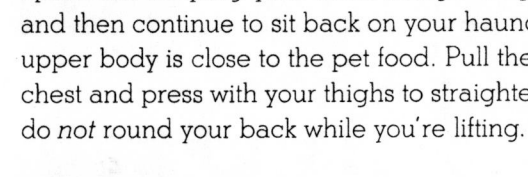

Mall Milers. Many malls open their hallways to morning walkers before the stores open. If your local weather makes you shudder when you consider walking outside, investigate whether your local mall has a walking program. Think of all the money you'll save by walking the mall while the stores are closed!

Pet-Food Squats. Whether or not you have a pet, squat down in the pet-food section and pick up a 10-pound sack of dry food. Do this without stressing your back or knees by standing with your legs wide apart and keeping your back straight as you bend your knees and then continue to sit back on your haunches until your whole upper body is close to the pet food. Pull the bag in close to your chest and press with your thighs to straighten up. Do not, do not, do *not* round your back while you're lifting.

Dentist Drill. You know the drill: You get to the dentist's or doctor's office right on time, only to be told they're "running a little late." If you can pin the receptionist down to a range of how many minutes you might be expected to wait, use that time to walk the hallway or walk around the block rather than reading those magazines from 1997. Tell the receptionist where you're going, and be sure to get back within plenty of time.

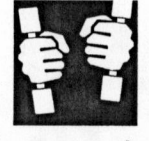 **Shopping Cart Curls.** Before it gets too full to lift, do biceps curls with the cart. Hold on to the handle with both hands, palms up, keeping your elbows in close to your waist. Bring your hands (and the cart handle) up toward your shoulders. Release slowly (and, we hope, without attracting too much attention). Do not try this when the cart is full of groceries or when a child is sitting in it, and do not try this with someone else's cart!

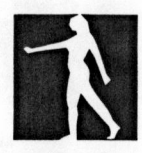 **Top-Shelf Reach.** Use a visit to the store as an excuse to stretch. Reach for an item on the top shelf (whether or not you really want it), bring it down, examine it, and return it to the top shelf. Switch arms and repeat with another item.

Aisle Aerobics. Don't waste time comparing brands of aspirin while you're waiting for your prescription to be ready. Use the time to powerwalk the store or hospital, walking the aisles or hallway as quickly as you can. A 150-pound person walking at a 3-mile-per-hour pace burns 3.75 calories a minute. Increasing the pace to 3.5 miles per hour pumps up calorie burning to 4.3 calories per minute. And if you have to wait 20 minutes for your prescription, that's a whole aerobic workout.

Shopping for Weight Loss

Is it really worth shifting your errand routine so it takes more time and makes you walk from store to store and up and down aisles, carrying heavy baskets or doing weird things with your shopping cart? The answer is a resounding "Yes!" whether you're increasing your activity for health (remember that accumulating a half hour a day is all you need) or increased energy (just get your heart rate up for a few minutes, and you'll feel invigorated).

If you're exercising with the goal of losing weight, remember that a 3,500-calorie deficit equals 1 pound of weight loss. To lose a pound, you need to burn 3,500 calories more than you eat. You won't accomplish this in a week just by making your errands more active—unless errands are a central focus of your day—but just 30 minutes of "active errands" twice a week can help you drop 4 pounds a year, and that's not even counting the activities you're doing the rest of the week.

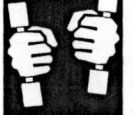 **Calf Line-Up.** Do one-legged calf raises whenever you have to wait in line: Stand on one leg, slowly push up onto the ball of your foot, and then slowly lower down. You'll strengthen your calves and—if you don't lean on the shopping cart—your abdominals. If you're having trouble balancing, let the lifted foot barely touch down with one toe to help stabilize you.

Errand Energizers

93

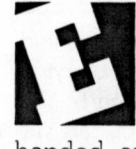 **Unload Yourself.** Move your own purchases from the shopping cart onto the cashier's platform instead of waiting for the cashier to do it. You'll burn 7½ times as many calories as standing there empty-handed, and you'll get through the line faster.

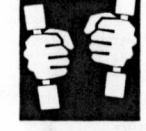 **Grocery Galvanizer.** If you're not picking up a cart-load of items, don't even use a cart. Carry a basket and perform biceps curls as you shop: Keep your elbow at your waist as you lift the basket up until your hand is close to shoulder height. Switch arms frequently.

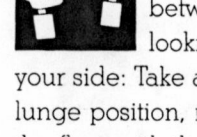 **Basket Lunge.** Better than carrying a basket is carrying two baskets, so you can distribute the weight between both sides of your body. When no one is looking, do a walking lunge holding your baskets at your side: Take a long step forward with the right foot. Sink into a lunge position, right knee over the ankle, left knee bent close to the floor with the heel up. Keep your back neutral. Push up and repeat with the left foot stepping forward. This exercise strengthens the thighs and buttocks.

 **Flights of Groceries.** If you have stairs to climb with your groceries, so much the better. Carrying groceries upstairs burns three times as many calories as carrying them on flat ground—and five times as many as sitting and watching someone else carry them!

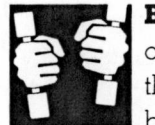 **Be a Bag Boy or Bag Lady.** Forget rolling the grocery cart to your car. Pick up your bags and carry them. Help some elderly shoppers by carrying their bags (with their permission). If you do use a shopping cart, return it to the store from the parking lot, and pick up any additional carts you find on the way.

Pal Play

Do you have a friend who might enjoy combining her or his errands with yours and doing them together? Tell your pal about your intention to make your errand-running as active as possible (even better, buy a copy of this book for your friend), and as you shop together, look for additional ways to be active. You'll get a few laughs and discover new activities that fit right in. (E-mail your best ideas to the author at joan@joanprice.com, please!)

Errand Energizers

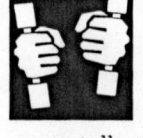 **Park the Remote.** When you get home, open the garage door manually instead of using the remote opener. You'll burn more than three times as many calories and get some strength-training besides, especially if your garage door is difficult to open.

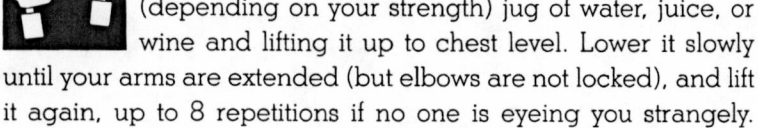 **Run Someone Else's Errands.** You're fortunate that you have a healthy, active body and can do the activities described in this chapter. You probably know a friend, neighbor, or relative who isn't so fortunate. Offer to do that person's errands, either on a regular basis or, if that's unrealistic with your schedule, spontaneously when you have a little extra time. You'll do a good deed, feel good about it, and, as a fringe benefit, get extra exercise.

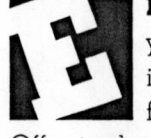 **Jug Lifts.** Strengthen your upper back in the grocery store by holding a gallon or half-gallon (depending on your strength) jug of water, juice, or wine and lifting it up to chest level. Lower it slowly until your arms are extended (but elbows are not locked), and lift it again, up to 8 repetitions if no one is eyeing you strangely. Keep your shoulders down throughout.

12

Chapter 8

9

Park
Pep-Ups

3

6

YOUR NEIGHBORHOOD PARK is an ideal place for minutes or hours of exercise. It's outdoors, combining a natural, open space with the energy of active people enjoying physical exercise, from kids climbing jungle gyms, swinging, and playing soccer, to grownups of all ages walking with friends and dogs, jogging, biking, and skating. A park can be a quieting place for you to be alone with your thoughts and nature or an opportunity to meet friends and enjoy lively, physical activity together.

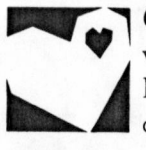

Getting There. If you live or work close enough, walk, don't drive, to the park. Stride, don't meander. If the park isn't within walking distance, how about driving almost there and walking the rest of the way?

Get Off Your Rocker. Sit on a park bench. Get up. Sit down again. Get up. Sit down. Get up. Exhale and pull in your abdominals as you rise, and keep your back neutral. Repeat 10 to 40 times, depending on your strength and stamina. If you have trouble getting up, put one foot in front of the other and "rock" onto the front foot to start the movement. Keep your eyes on a point directly in front of you instead of looking down, because your body will go where you're looking, and if you look down at the ground, it will be harder to get up from the sitting position. This exercise strengthens the quadriceps (front of your thighs) and abdominals. It can also get your heart rate up if you keep a steady rhythm and don't stop to rest.

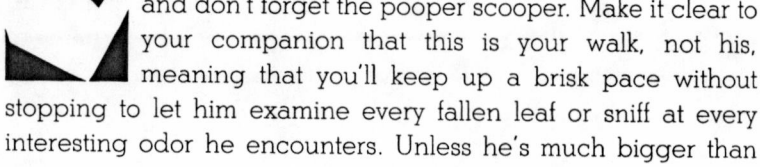

Walk a Dog. Take your favorite canine to the park, and don't forget the pooper scooper. Make it clear to your companion that this is your walk, not his, meaning that you'll keep up a brisk pace without stopping to let him examine every fallen leaf or sniff at every interesting odor he encounters. Unless he's much bigger than you are, encourage him to break into a run, then pace yourself to keep up. If you don't have your own, offer to walk the neighbor's dog. The neighbor will owe you a favor, and you'll burn calories, more if the dog is young, speedy, and determined. Here's a social advantage for singles: Potential dates who won't look at you in a coffeehouse or on a bus may melt and make a fuss over your handsome hound.

Pooch Play. If you're allowed to let your dog off the leash in your park, play active games with her. Throw a ball or stick for her to catch. Don't just stand there waiting for her return—run yourself and let her chase you. Be careful that your dog is obedient and trained for such wild play before you go all-out, though, because dogs can get overexcited and accidentally knock you down (or, worse, knock down a passerby). If you're not sure, practice in your own yard before taking this dog-and-owner show on the road.

Bench Push-Ups. Do push-ups with your feet on the ground, your hands on a park bench. Make your body as long as possible, keeping your abdominals tight and your body in a straight line—no sinking at the stomach or hips. Bend your elbows to lower your body, then straighten your arms to raise it again. Do not lock your elbows.

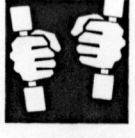 **Macho Bench Push-Ups.** Advanced only: If full Bench Push-Ups are a cinch for you, put your hands on the ground and your feet up on the bench, your hands and toes taking your weight. Now do your push-ups! Be sure to keep your back neutral and your abs tight. Lead with your chest, not your chin, nose, or belly.

Waist Whittlers

If your park has a board for abdominals, use it; otherwise, lie on a park bench or on the grass, knees bent, feet flat. This series works the abs in different ways.

1. **Slow Crunch.** Cross your arms on your chest or hold your head lightly in your hands. Watching the sky, contract the abdominal muscles, exhaling, and let that contraction lift the chest up to the count of 3 until the shoulders (or, if you're strong enough, the shoulder blades) are slightly raised. Hold at the top for 3 seconds, breathing normally. Then take 4 seconds to lower down. Repeat 4 times.
2. **Fast Crunch.** Do **Slow Crunch** (above) but faster: up for 2 seconds and down for 2 seconds, repeating 8 times.
3. **Alternating Crunches.** Do one **Slow Crunch** and 2 **Fast Crunches**, repeating the combination 4 times.
4. **Twists.** Lift up as if you're doing a **Slow Crunch**, but then twist at the waist, aiming one shoulder toward the opposite knee. Do 4 to one side, then 4 to the other, then alternate for 4.

100 After working the abdominals, do the **Grassy Low-Back Stretch** (p. 101).

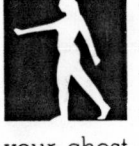 **Bench Dip.** Sit on the edge of a park bench (facing away from the table, if there is a table), hands on the edge of the bench, knuckles toward your body. Now shift your weight off the bench so that your derrière is a few inches in front of the bench and unsupported. Your body is supported only by your hands on the bench and feet on the ground. Alternate bending your elbows and straightening your arms, lowering and raising your body. Be careful not to let your shoulders hunch—keep them pushed down. Your triceps (back of the upper arms) are doing the work. Make this more difficult by walking your feet out farther away from the bench—now your weight is more on your arms than your legs.

Grassy Low-Back Stretch. Lie down on a flat spot on the grass, knees bent, feet flat. Bring the legs up, wrapping your arms around your thighs, hands clasped (if you can reach). Pull your thighs in toward your chest, stretching your lower back. Hold for 10 to 60 seconds.

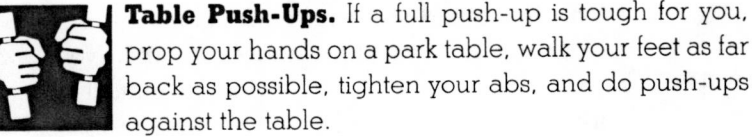 **Table Push-Ups.** If a full push-up is tough for you, prop your hands on a park table, walk your feet as far back as possible, tighten your abs, and do push-ups against the table.

Tree Push-Away, Beginner: The easiest upper-body strengthener is an upright "push-away." Stand about an arm's length away from a tree, palms flat on the tree at chest height and a little wider than shoulder width. (A skinny tree won't work.) Keeping your body in a line as if you were in a body cast, bend your elbows, letting your body bend from the ankles (lift the heels) until your nose is close enough to smell the bark. Exhale and push yourself up to standing again. Repeat 8 to 12 times.

Wind Sprints. Walk the park, alternating between a steady, moderate pace and little intervals at a faster pace. Your goal is to push your limits a bit with bursts of speed, but not to the point of getting out of breath. Make the speed intervals very brief at first—just 5 to 10 seconds of speed for every 5 minutes or so at a slower, comfortable pace. Later on, as you get more conditioned, you can work up to longer speed intervals and do them more frequently. You can make a game of this by racing to the next tree or resting in the shade and speedwalking in the sun.

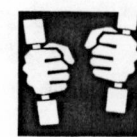

Tree Sit. Stand with your back against a sturdy and fairly straight tree trunk, and slowly inch your way partway down, keeping your back in contact with the tree. Walk your feet away from the tree so they stay right under your knees, until your thighs are taking your weight and you look like you're sitting in an invisible chair with the tree trunk as your backrest. Hold that pose, breathing normally, until your thighs tell you to get up—it won't take long!

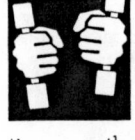

Pull-Down Stretch. If your park has a pull-up station—a high, horizontal bar for doing pull-ups or chin-ups—don't skip it just because you're not strong enough to chin yourself. Instead, use it for a great upper-body stretch. Grab the horizontal bar and let your body weight sink until—depending on your height and the height of the bar—you're either really hanging from the bar (your feet are off the ground) or practically hanging (your toes are still on the ground, but most of your weight is hanging from the bar). If the bar is too short for either of these positions, bend your knees as if you'd kneel on the ground if you could get low enough, but you can't. Whichever position you end up in, you'll feel a super stretch through the back, shoulders, and arms.

Station Stops. Some parks have exercise "stations" with some sort of apparatus and a sign explaining how to use it. For example, there might be a pull-up pole, or footrests for a hamstring stretch, or rubber tires on the ground to run. Explore whatever stations your park has, and feel free to experiment with other ways to use them.

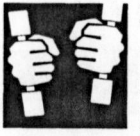 **Pole Pulls.** Stand with your knees on either side of the pole of a signpost, holding on with both hands. Lean back away from the pole in a seated position (derrière back, knees bent), as if you had a chair behind you (which you don't), letting your body weight pull away from the pole. Pretend that you're pulling the pole toward your chest (you're actually pulling your chest toward the pole), elbows back, squeezing the shoulder blades as the pole gets close to your chest. Repeat 8 times slowly. This works the large muscles of the back.

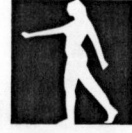 **Tree Hug.** After working the back muscles with the **Pole Pulls** above, a back stretch will feel just dandy. Find a slim tree (or a thick, low-hanging branch) that you can get your arms around, and hang back, knees bent, back rounded. Hold for 10 to 60 seconds, depending on how good it makes your back feel and how comfortable it is to hold on to the tree.

Park Socials

If you're dashing to the park for a quick pick-me-up, you'll do fine on your own. But if you have 1 hour or an entire afternoon, it's nice to let the park be the venue for some socializing with your friends or a date. Here are some ideas to get you started.

- Instead of making a lunch date with a friend, pack sandwiches or get some healthy deli takeout, and meet your friend in the park.

Walk and talk, enjoying the fresh air and the feeling of your muscles moving as well as the pleasure of your friend's company. Then settle in a shady spot to eat your lunch.

- Organize an active sport at the park with friends or family on a weekend afternoon. Depending on your park's resources, your time, and your preferences, you might plan Frisbee, volleyball, softball, bicycling, inline skating, or a hike.
- We all have old friends whom we see too seldom. Invite an old friend to meet you at the park, and catch up by exchanging news as you walk and stretch.
- Single folks generally find first dates ghastly (until, of course, you meet Mr./ Ms. Right or Right Now). Instead of sitting through an interminable dinner, or chatting over too much caffeine at a coffee shop, or staring at a movie and not talking at all, plan your first date at the park. You can get to know each other by talking as you walk the park. And if the date's a dud, at least you got your exercise.

Calf Stretch. Stand close to a tree or fence, facing it, and push against it with both hands. Step back with the right leg and press the heel down. The left leg is slightly bent. Feel the stretch in the right calf. Then bring the right leg forward a couple of inches and slightly bend the right knee, feeling the stretch go lower in the calf. Hold for 10 to 60 seconds. Repeat with the other leg.

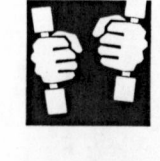

Monkey Bar Antics. Remember how we used to travel the monkey bars with such ease when we were kids? Try it now: Climb up, grab hold of the closest top bar, and swing your body as you alternate hands grabbing the next bar until you're all the way across. This is much more effort for a grownup than for a kid, so be prepared!

Monkey Bar Antics, Modified. If you're not strong enough to traverse the bars, try a few pull-ups from the first bar. When you're tired, drop down, and be sure to stretch your back before leaving.

Hamstring (back of thigh) Stretch. Stand at your favorite scenic spot. Extend the right leg straight in front of you, foot flexed (toes up), the left leg slightly bent. Lean the upper body forward from the hips, hands on thighs. (You can hold on to a fence or tree if it's more comfortable). Lower your body and push your weight away from your right foot, bending your left leg and pushing your derrière back until you feel a pleasurable stretch in the back of the right thigh. Hold for 10 to 60 seconds. Switch sides.

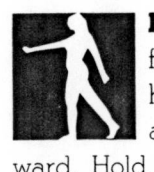 **Back Fence Chest Stretch.** If your park has a sturdy fence that permits you to face away from it and still hold on securely, hold onto the fence behind you at about hip height (if you have a choice) and lean forward. Hold for 10 to 60 seconds. You'll get a nice chest and shoulder stretch.

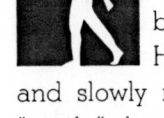 **Quad (front of thigh) Stretch.** Stand close to a fence or tree, facing it, and push against it with the right hand. Reach back with the left hand and bend the left knee until you can hold on to your left ankle (or sock or pant leg) behind you. Try to align the thighs and straighten the back, feeling the stretch in the front of the left thigh. Hold for 10 to 60 seconds. Repeat with the other leg.

Mid-Back Stretch. Hold on to a fence, slender tree, or pole, facing it. Round your back, pulling your body weight away from the object you're holding. Hold for 10 to 60 seconds, then slowly straighten up, and slowly round down into position again. Feel the stretch "ripple" through your back muscles while you're moving, and feel your muscles relax while you're holding the stretch.

Park Pep-Ups

107

12

Chapter 9

9   Getting It   3
Together:
Making
Exercise Fun

6

W HAT'S THE BEST EXERCISE FOR YOU? The one you'll do!
The best way you can become an active person is to
find types of movement that you genuinely look forward to doing. Whether you want to stick to little spurts of
exercise throughout the day, create a full-fledged exercise
habit, play a favorite sport, enjoy active leisure activities, or
some combination of these, your choices must be enjoyable
for you, personally.

There's no single best choice for everybody. Health clubs
are perfect for some people and torment for others. Some
people are happy gardening and miserable lifting weights.   **109**

Other people live to dance and can't imagine getting on a treadmill. Some delight in practical activity—remodeling the kitchen, washing the car, painting the house—and would be bored to tears walking without anyplace to go.

You need to look at what would make *you* feel comfortable easing into exercise—this book is a terrific start!—and which activities give you a smile and a feeling of satisfaction. Once you find some physical activities that you really enjoy, exercise will become a treat (not a treatment) and a highlight of your day, not a chore. Your fitness program will only work if you've chosen the right activities for your goals, preferences, and lifestyle—and if you enjoy it. These tips—and the activities all the way through this book—will help you discover the fun in fitness.

But I Hate Exercise!

If you think exercise is torture, you haven't found the right type for you. Realize that exercise, for you, might not be an aerobics video, or jogging, or any of the common activities that we think of as "exercise." If you've never thought that "exercise" and "joy" fit in the same thought, try this: Brainstorm a list of activities requiring physical exertion (we don't have to call it "exercise") that you would enjoy doing. Jitterbugging, gardening, playing catch with the kids, canoeing, horseback riding, shooting hoops, swimming, building a deck—you name it. Stretch your mind to find activities that bring a smile to your face. See if you can indulge one of these activities this weekend.

Revisit the Past

If you're stumped trying to find exercise options that you enjoy, look at a sport or other activity you used to find fun, but somehow left behind. Make a list of physical activities you used to enjoy as a child, teenager, or young adult, and see how you can bring one of those back into your life. Did you enjoy bicycling? Skating? Swimming? Volleyball? Hula-Hoops? Frisbee? Rock 'n' roll dancing? You can do all these again (well, maybe not the Hula-Hoop),and you'll probably enjoy them just as much now!

===== **Personality Match** =====

You're more likely to stick with an activity program if it fits your personality. Which type describes you, and which activities fit your type?

- **You like to compete:** Choose an active sport with a "winner," such as tennis, volleyball, basketball, soccer, or racquetball.
- **You enjoy social interaction:** Choose social dance, golf with friends (no golf cart!), group hikes, group bicycling, health clubs, exercise classes, mall walking, or ice skating at a rink.
- **You want to be out in nature:** Choose an outdoor activity like hiking, water or snow skiing, horseback riding, beach running, or walking.

- **You enjoy getting things done:** Garden, mow the lawn, wash the car, do carpentry or housework.
- **You're a loner:** Exercise in the privacy of your home, take a walk in the park, hike a trail, bicycle, exercise to a video, swim, or do t'ai chi, yoga, or martial arts.
- **You're goal oriented:** Try traditional fitness activities that let you track your progress, such as logging how fast you run, how far you walk, how much you lift, or how many miles you bicycle.

Mix It Up

You'd go nuts if you ate the same food or had the same conversations every day. Your exercise activities need variety, too. Keep stimulating your muscles and your mind with change. Maybe bicycle the first day, walk the next, and garden the next. Organize some friends for a weekend outing at the park. Make time for a hike or a swim. If you've been lifting weights, go for a walk. Try a new exercise video. Take a dance class. The possibilities are limited only by your imagination and open-mindedness. The point is to make exercise a habit that you look forward to, and variety is the key.

Try Something Brand New

If you've never tried line dancing, you can't imagine how much fun it is. Ditto for mountain biking, beach volleyball, hiking to see the wildflowers—who knows what new activity you'd really enjoy? Ask your friends and colleagues what they enjoy, and let them introduce you to their favorite activities. You might find a new activity that opens a whole new world to you.

Choosing and Using Exercise Videotapes

The advantages of exercise videotapes are many. You can work out at any hour you choose, in any weather, and in private. You can wear your oldest sweats or your husband's boxer shorts if you wish. You can keep an eye on the kids and be there to answer the phone. You can start and stop the tape as many times as you want to learn a routine, call the instructor nasty names, or even say no and turn her off. You don't have to do the whole workout—you can exercise for 5, 30, or 11½ minutes, or whatever you please. You're in control of the "start," "stop," and "pause" controls! Best of all, exercise videos are fun. You're working out with some of the best instructors in the country, who know how to design a terrific workout and motivate you to do it.

Aerobic dance videotapes are the best known, but you can enjoy any kind of exercise with a videotape: step, strength training, yoga, Pilates, and kickboxing, for example. You can find specialty workouts for special conditions, such as arthritis, back pain, or pregnancy—even workouts done in a chair. And if you're looking for a special focus, from ballet to belly dancing to swing dancing, you'll find it on videotape. A video is about the cheapest exercise tool you can buy for total-body fitness, ranging in price from $10 to $30, with most in the $15 to $20 range.

Only a few workout tapes are distributed in stores—those by celebrities and the big-name fitness professionals. Some of these are good, but you're choosing from just a few of the hundreds of exercise videos available by mail, Internet, or phone, which we recommend. (See the Resources Appendix for recommended sources of exercise videos.)

You can't judge an exercise video by its cover—or by its cover girl. One best-selling exercise videotape, for example, was a popular model's unsafe workout, which was panned by every credible fitness professional who saw it and which one exercise expert called a "chiropractor's nightmare." So don't choose a video just because the leader looks good—look for her or his credentials.

If buying from a store, read the back of the box. If buying online or from a mail-order catalog, read the reviews carefully. Here's what you're looking for:

- **What are the leader's or consultant's credentials?** The best workouts are not celebrity videos, but those that feature certified fitness instructors who have spent their professional lives learning about exercise effectiveness, safety, and teaching methods and perfecting their skills over decades of teaching real people in real classes. Sometimes the leader is not certified but is assisted by a consultant who is certified, has an exercise science degree, or is a medical professional. This consultant may have designed and supervised the workout off-camera or may be on-camera demonstrating the moves with the leader.

- **What does the workout include?** Does the description match the claim on the front cover? For example, if it claims to "burn fat," the workout must be aerobic. You can usually find a breakdown of the different sections, such as the warm-up, the different segments of the workout, and the cool-down/stretch, including the number of minutes of each, on the back cover or in a review. You're looking for a workout that will fit your goals and your schedule: long enough to be effective, but not so long that you won't do it.

- **What ability level does it target?** Select a video designed for your level. Some workouts are multilevel because they include modifications for making the moves easier or harder; but if this isn't stated, don't expect it. If you're just starting a program, look for a tape that specifies beginning level.

- **When was the videotape made?** Look for more recent videos, because safety guidelines have changed over the years, and instructors know more now about how to design an effective workout. Be aware that older videos are often reissued as new ones, yet nothing has changed except the cover art. Read the small print on the box, and look for that information in reviews.

- **What equipment do you need?** Some videos require equipment or tools such as weights, a step, or bands. The box or review should tell you.

If you discover that videos work for you, get a few so you can switch around according to your mood, energy level, and preference. For all-around fitness, include aerobics, strength training, and flexibility. (Be sure to read Chapter 17 before exercising with a workout video. See the Resources Appendix to learn where to order exercise videos.)

=========== **Every Step Counts** ===========

Why do so many of the exercises in this book involve walking? Walking is the simplest form of "portable" exercise for most of us—we can do it anywhere, anytime, whether we're running errands, traveling, socializing, or seeking solitude. It's one of the healthiest and most enjoyable physical activities, requiring no equipment, props, or special clothing. You can decide on the spur of the moment to walk, with no preparation.

If you're working on accumulating enough walking for health benefits, an alternative to counting exercise minutes is to track your steps. Don't worry, you won't have to carry a calculator or compulsively count every step aloud. We recommend wearing a pedometer—a gadget smaller than a pager that clips to your belt or waistband and counts every time you take a step. This is not only a great way to track your daily activity—it's a cool tool that will inspire you to move more so you can see the steps add up. Plus, the pedometer adds an extra element of fun and a feeling of success in reaching goals. (See the Resources Appendix for more information about where to find pedometers.)

For health benefits, try to take 10,000 steps a day, a level determined by Stanford University and the Cooper Institute for Aerobics Research. That sounds like a lot, but if you're active in the way we recommend in this book, you'll make it. Just going about your business without trying to incorporate any physical activity, you will probably take about 3,000 to 4,000 steps a day, depending on how often you pop up out of your chair. So you just need to add an extra 6,000 to 7,000, which you can do with the kinds of activities you'll find in this book, to total 10,000.

Ten thousand steps is roughly equivalent to walking 5 miles. That might seem like quite a distance, but you'll see how your daily activity steps add up if you wear the pedometer as you incorporate extra exercise minutes into your day. Taking 10,000 steps a day will burn between 2,000 and 3,500 extra calories per week—enough to lose a pound of body fat.

Lose Your Job

Try an exercise activity that is very different from what you do at work. For example, if your job is demanding and time-pressured, get outside and hike in the woods or walk the beach, and feel your tension evaporate. If your job is task-oriented and full of details, you might like a cardio machine, which allows you to zone out and not concentrate on anything. If you feel like you can't express your individuality at work, choose an activity where you can really break loose and express yourself, like dancing or kickboxing. If you're held back at work, you might like exercise that lets you take off at a fast pace, like cycling or running. If you're surrounded by other people's demands all day, you might enjoy solitary exercise with no one telling you what to do, like swimming or hiking. And if you resent the time you spend away from home when you're working, you might be happy with a home-based program like gardening, walking the dog, and working out at home to an exercise video.

Let the Music Play

Music can enhance any type of workout—not just aerobic dance—and motivate you to go a little longer and maybe a little more intensely. Whatever physical activity you're doing—push-ups, housecleaning, chopping wood, crunches—play a selection of favorite, upbeat music that makes you want to move.

12

Chapter 10

9   **At Home:**   3
   Before Dinner

6

WHAT DO YOU USUALLY DO when you first get home from work? Unwind with the newspaper and a glass of wine? Watch the news? Start making dinner? Sort through the mail? Get the children started on their homework? Wish that you had time to exercise? However crushed your time seems, you'll actually have more time in the evening if you work some physical activity into your transition time. This is because you'll energize your body and mind instead of sinking into fatigue, and you'll find you can enjoy your evening more. Here are some ideas you can work into the pre-dinner hour—some of them can be done even while you're cooking!

 **Bicycle Blitz.** The moment you arrive home, change to your bike shorts or sweats, grab your helmet, and mount your bike for a short ride. If you're an experienced cyclist, make that a fast-paced ride. You'll work off stress, energize for the evening, and burn calories at the rate of 5 to 13 a minute, depending on speed and terrain. Wear reflective clothing and lights if you're doing this after dark. Advanced: Make that a fast-paced, *hilly* ride. Feel free to substitute riding a stationary bike if you don't have a road bike or if the weather sends you back indoors. A 150-pound person cycling for just 15 minutes will burn 136 calories at 12 to 13.9 miles per hour (moderate speed) or 170 calories at 14 to 15.9 miles per hour (fast, vigorous effort). Adding hills revs up the calorie burning substantially, depending on how hard the climb.

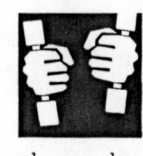 **Tea Kettle Lifts.** Fill your tea kettle under the faucet, then lift and lower the kettle by raising and lowering your hand at the wrist, keeping your arm steady. This strengthens the wrist. Do 8 to 12 repetitions, then change hands.

 **Jump Off Pounds.** If you jump rope for 10 minutes instead of playing sofa spud while you watch the evening news each weekday, you can burn off 11 pounds in a year.

Dog Walk. If you live in the country or have a fenced yard, it's easy just to open the door and let Poochie out to do his business. But if you let Poochie take you for a 30-minute walk instead, you'll burn 125 calories (contrasted with 2 calories to open the door to let out the dog), and your pup will be grateful and much healthier, too.

The Perfect Crunch

This basic crunch, recommended by Bryant Stamford, Ph.D., director of the Health Promotion and Wellness Center and professor of exercise physiology at the University of Louisville, will strengthen your abs and back. Pay careful attention to your form and technique to get the most benefits from this abdominal workhorse.

1. Lie on your back, knees bent. Your hands can be crossed on your chest, relaxed beside your head, relaxed at your side, or crossed behind your head. Do not interlace your fingers behind your head—this makes it too easy to pull on your head.
2. Contract your abdominal muscles as you exhale. Focus on the contraction, imagining it pulling your rib cage toward your hipbone.
3. Let the contraction pull your shoulders, chest, and shoulder blades up slowly off the floor. Do not use momentum or pull on your head with your hands.

4. Pause when your upper body is about halfway to an upright position (about 6 to 12 inches off the floor) and hold the contraction for a moment. Beginners: Don't worry if you can't get that high—it's enough to feel the contraction, even if you get just 1 inch off the floor.
5. Lower *slowly* to the floor, resisting gravity's pull, inhaling.
6. Do not relax when your head touches the floor. Tighten the contraction and begin again. Continue until fatigued.

Advanced: If you can do 20 of these crunches slowly and in good form, make them harder by adding resistance. Hold dumbbells on your chest, by your ears, or behind your head. The farther away the weight is from your abs, the harder the crunch. Don't anchor your feet under a chair—that's cheating! And don't think you're working your abs harder if you come all the way up—then you're working your hip flexors instead and stressing your back.

Counter Levitations. Advanced only: If you're strong enough to do push-ups barely trembling, try this on a sturdy kitchen counter. Lean over the kitchen counter, hands flat, elbows bent. Straighten your back, bend your knees, and cross your feet at the ankles. Push yourself straight up, using your triceps (back of the upper arms), bending your knees more, until your feet leave the floor. Hold, slowly release. Repeat until your triceps scream or until your counter collapses, whichever comes first.

Dance the Day Away. As soon as you come into the house, change to comfortable clothes, turn on your favorite style of "gotta move!" music, and boogie down. Dance around the room in whatever style fits your mood of the moment. Sing along if you're so inspired. If you're self-conscious about dancing, you can substitute jumping jacks or running around the living room.

Run the Stairs. You can get a great cardio workout just going up and down (and up and down) a flight of stairs at a brisk pace. Don't go so fast that you get winded, but push yourself so that you're in your aerobic zone. Warm up by climbing the stairs at a normal pace first. Be sure you're wearing nonslip shoes. Advanced: Run up the stairs and walk down.

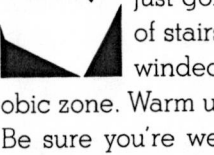

Dyna-Band Two-Somes. You don't have time for a full-body strength-training workout? No problem. While dinner cooks, choose one muscle group and its opposing group, and train them with Dyna-Bands. (Note: These exercises are based on the presumption that you have the recommended two pairs, a pair each at two different intensities, so that you can work your stronger muscles with the harder bands and your weaker muscles with the easier bands. See the Resources

Appendix for more information.) Do 8 to 12 slow repetitions of your choice of the following exercises, pairing them by opposing muscle groups (chest and back, biceps and triceps, quadriceps and hamstrings). Add the shoulder exercises when you have 1 extra minute.

- **Back.** Sit on the floor, the middle of your hardest band anchored around the soles of your feet, knees apart. Cross the band in front of your legs so that you're holding opposite ends. Pull the elbows back until your hands come to your ribs, as if you're rowing, and squeeze your shoulder blades at the end of the move. Release slowly. Keep your back straight and shoulders down throughout the move. Repeat. Advanced: If even your hardest band is too easy for these large muscles, double up and use both of your strongest bands together.

- **Chest.** Put the hardest band around the middle of your back, bringing the ends out under your arms until they're in front of you at chest level. Hold the band so that the ends come under your thumbs and over your hands. Push your arms straight out in front of you, keeping your shoulders down, your chest up, and not locking the elbows. You can cross your hands slightly at the end for more intensity. Repeat. Advanced: If even your hardest band is too easy for these large muscles, double up and use both of your strongest bands together.

- **Biceps** *(front of upper arm)*. Stand with your heels anchoring the ends of a pair of easier bands, with just a bit of each end showing between your feet. Hold the other ends of the band wrapped around your hands at your side, palms up, so that there is some tension in the band even when your arms are relaxed. Keeping your elbows at your waist, bring your hands toward your shoulders, being careful to keep your back neutral and still. Repeat.
- **Triceps** *(back of upper arm)*. Hold one of your easier bands overhead with the right hand, elbow bent and pointing to the ceiling, not sticking out to the side. Grasp the lower part of the band with the left hand behind your back at waist level. Anchor the left hand either behind your back or at your side, whichever is more comfortable. Slowly straighten the right arm above your head, being careful to keep the wrist straight, knuckles up, until your arm is straight, the band is stretched, and your triceps are trembling. Slowly bend—don't let the band snap down—and repeat. If this seems too easy, shorten the amount of band between your hands for the full exercise. Change arms after your set of 8 to 12 repetitions.
- **Shoulders.** Stand with your heels anchoring the ends of two easier bands, with just a bit of each end showing between your feet. Hold the other ends of the bands in front of your hipbones, with slight tension in the bands, elbows slightly bent, thumbs up. Open the arms and lift the elbows until

your upper arms, elbows, and lower arms are all at shoulder height. Be careful to keep your elbows slightly bent, back straight, and shoulders down. Repeat.

- **Quadriceps** *(front of thigh)* **and Buttocks.** Stand with your heels on the ends of two harder bands, with just a bit of each end showing between your feet. Bring the other ends up behind your back and over your shoulders, gripping the ends at your shoulders. Sit back as if you had a chair behind you, keeping your back neutral and your chest up. Keep your weight over your heels, not letting your knees come forward of your toes. Squeeze your buttock muscles as you straighten up. Repeat.

- **Hamstrings** *(back of thigh).* Tie one end of one easier band around one foot. Hold on to a chair and stand so that the heel of your other foot anchors the band about 8 to 10 inches in front of the tied foot. Raise the tied foot behind you by bending your knee, then slowly lower. Repeat the whole set with one leg before changing to the other. For more information about Dyna-Bands, see the Resources Appendix.

"Just Say No" to Phone Solicitors. Don't you hate the way phone marketers always call at dinner time? Release the stress in your neck when you answer by slowly turning your head from side to side, like you're gesturing "No." Hang up, and do a couple more slow head turns.

Dyna-Band Crunches

You can also use a Dyna-Band to make your abdominal workout harder on your abs and easier on your neck. Place your hardest band full-length on the rug or mat. Sit so that one end is right under your tailbone. Then, keeping knees bent and feet flat, lie down on top of the band so that your spine is along the length of the band. Reach behind your head to grip the top end with both hands, and pull it beyond your head, stretching the band into a "hammock" for your head. (Be sure you don't dig your nails into the band—that can rip it.) Your head should rest on the band comfortably. Take a deep breath. As you exhale, pull your abdominal muscles in and let that muscle contraction lift your chest, then shoulders, then—if you're strong enough—shoulder blades. Let your head rest—don't pull on it. Hold at the top for 2 seconds before slowly releasing down. Keep your head and neck relaxed through the whole sequence. Repeat 8 to 12 times or more.

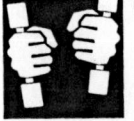 **Push Your Rug.** Do 8 to 12 repetitions of either straight-leg or bent-knee push-ups on your living room rug. Keep your hands under your shoulders or a little wider. Keep your body rigid, as if you were in a body cast, with your head, neck, and spine in alignment and the abdominals contracted. (If you're doing bent-leg push-ups, keep your weight a little forward of your knees, on the padded parts between your knees and thighs, not on your kneecaps. Raise your feet and cross them.) Lead with the chest—don't dip the chin or forehead. Go slowly: no faster than 2 seconds down and 2 seconds up, even slower if

you're strong. Exhale on the way up. Be careful to keep your abdominals tight and your back neutral. Don't let your hips or belly sag.

Refrigerator Push-Away. If full push-ups are too difficult, here's a modification. Stand facing the refrigerator, a little more than arm's length away. Brace your hands against the fridge and bend your elbows. Your body will be on a slant now from head (close to the refrigerator) to heels. Keeping your abdominals tight and your body aligned (not sagging, arching, or rounding), push with your arms as if you're pushing the refrigerator away (symbolic, yes?). When your arms are straight but not locked, bend again. Repeat 8 to 12 times, exhaling as you push. This strengthens the chest and arms and prevents you from opening the refrigerator, at least while you're doing the exercise.

Chop Your Own. Those prewashed, prechopped veggies are convenient, and we recommend them when you don't have the time or inclination to prepare your own. But realize that if you wash, slice, or chop vegetables yourself for 15 minutes, you burn 10 to 13 calories. That's a puny number compared to jogging or kickboxing, granted, but it's 10 to 13 times as many as buying your vegetables presliced or frozen. And your veggies will be fresher.

Fit Feet

Don't neglect your tootsies when keeping your body in shape. The following exercises are recommended by The American Orthopaedic Foot and Ankle Society (*www.aofas.org*) to keep your feet strong and flexible. They're especially good for dancers and runners, but also for regular folks whose feet spend most of the day in shoes.

- **Toe Raise, Toe Point, Toe Curl.** Push up onto the ball of one foot. Then point the foot, big toe touching the floor. Then curl the big toe under, toward the sole, and push into the floor with the "knuckle" of the toe. Hold each position for 5 seconds and repeat 10 times with each foot. Especially recommended for people with hammertoes or toe cramps.
- **Toe Pulls.** Put a thick rubber band around all of your toes and spread them. Hold this position for 5 seconds, then release. Repeat 10 times. Especially recommended for people with bunions, hammertoes, or toe cramps.
- **Golf Ball Roll.** Roll a golf ball under the ball of your foot for 2 minutes, massaging the bottom of your foot. Especially recommended for people with plantar fasciitis (heel pain), arch strain, or foot cramps.
- **Towel Curls.** Place a small towel on the floor and curl it toward you, using only your toes to bunch up the towel. You can make this harder by putting a weight on the end of the towel and pulling it toward you. Relax and repeat this exercise 5 times. Especially recommended for people with hammertoes, toe cramps, and pain in the ball of the foot.
- **Marble Pick-Up.** Place 20 marbles on the floor. Pick up one marble at a time by clutching it under your toes, and put it in a

small bowl. Repeat until you have picked up all 20 marbles. Especially recommended for people with pain in the ball of the foot, hammertoes, and toe cramps.

Balanced Nutrition. Are you heating a pot of soup or a casserole? While it's still cold, hold the pot or filled casserole dish with both hands. Pulling in your abdominals, slowly lift one knee so you are balancing on one leg. This is a thigh and abdominal strengthener. Advanced: Extend the lifted leg straight ahead of you, continuing to balance on the standing leg. Beginners: Practice without holding the casserole dish first.

Stirring Move #1. When you have to stand at the stove stirring something, stand with one foot on your thickest cookbook (lengthwise, not across the spine), the other foot suspended (not touching the book or the floor). Do one-legged squats with the standing leg by sitting back as if you were going to place your derrière in a chair behind you and then you change your mind and stand up again. Beginners: Touch the floor lightly with the dangling foot. Advanced: Don't touch the floor at all with the dangling foot. Repeat 5 times with one leg before switching legs. This is a very effective thigh and buttock strengthener using your body weight. You can do this when you're not stirring, too.

Stirring Move #2. Still standing with one foot on your thickest cookbook, do outer-thigh lifts with the suspended leg by pressing it out to the side, knee facing forward. Repeat 8 to 12 times slowly before switching legs. (Switch the stirring arm when you switch the lifting leg.)

Drawer Stretch. Hold on to the handles of side-by-side kitchen drawers. Walk your feet away, bending at the waist, until you're far enough away to feel a lovely stretch in your back, shoulders, and arms. If you don't have handled side-by-side kitchen drawers, you can rest your hands on the countertop or table instead.

Essential Stretches

Many people don't know which body parts are important to stretch, says Seattle-based exercise physiologist Alice Lockridge, M.S. Physical Education (*www.exercisexpress.com*), owner of Exercise Express, a personal training studio, and PRO©FIT, a fitness instructor training company. Here are her essential stretches, which target the areas where people are typically tight. Remember to hold stretches 10 to 60 seconds and do them when you are already warmed up.

- **Shoulder.** Lie on your back on the floor with your arms straight overhead, trying to touch the floor with your wrists. Keep your elbows straight, arms close to your head. Hold.

- **Back Rotation.** Lie on your back on the floor with arms out wide. Cross one leg over your body. Relax. Do the other side.
- **Back Diagonal.** Sit on the floor cross-legged (if comfortable). Lift the right arm overhead, leaning over to the left side, arm up and over at a diagonal. Imagine that you're holding keys in your hand; your arm should be far enough over to the side so that if you drop the keys, they won't land on your head.
- **Lower Back.** Sit on the floor, legs either out in front or cross-legged, hands on the floor. Round your back and bend forward.
- **Hamstring (back of thigh).** Lie on your back on the floor with your tailbone against a wall, legs up on the wall, bent as much as necessary for comfort. Straighten your legs slowly until you reach your limit. Hold and relax into the stretch.
- **Upper Calf (gastrocnemius).** Stand, holding on to a piece of furniture for balance. Put your right foot in front of you, pointing straight forward. Keep your heel down and step past it with the left foot, keep the right leg straight. Push your hips forward (away from your heel). Hold and repeat with the other leg.
- **Deeper Calf (soleus).** Do the same action as Upper Calf, but keep the front foot close and bend the back knee slightly.

Stretch after warming up, and hold for at least 10 seconds. If you're very tight, hold the stretch longer—1 minute or more—relaxing into it. To improve flexibility, stretch at the end of your workout and hold for at least 60 seconds. Stay at the point where there's no pain. Never bounce when you stretch.

12

Chapter 11

9 **At Home:** 3
Anytime

6

EXERCISING AT HOME IS EASY AND CONVENIENT, especially once you start seeing opportunities for fitting minutes of physical activity into the day. It's easy to strengthen and stretch at home, and you don't need special equipment. You can catch exercise opportunities in the morning, in the evening, on the weekend, between other responsibilities or leisure activities, or whenever the mood strikes you. Try squeezing a few of these exercises into your at-home time, most using just stairs, furniture, and ordinary household items. Many of these quickies take less than 1 minute each. How many can you do in 1 day?

(See also the other "at home" chapters—Chapter 3 and Chapter 10—for more ideas for home-based activities. Many of the exercises in Chapter 16 can also be done at home.)

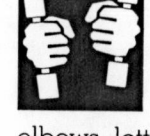 **Phone Sprints.** When the phone rings, don't reach for the closest extension. Run for the one farthest away, preferably up or down a flight of stairs. Set the answering machine to pick up in four rings so you have to hurry. Running upstairs burns fifteen times as many calories as sitting down and picking up the telephone.

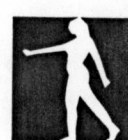 **Doorway Push-Away.** Stand in a doorway, one palm pressing against each side at about chest level. Walk back until your arms are almost straight. Still pressing your palms against the doorway, bend the elbows, letting your body fall forward (your heels lift off the floor), then press with your arms against the doorway to bring you back to standing position. Repeat 8 to 12 times. This works the chest and shoulders.

Doorway Back Stretch. Stand in a doorway, hands gripping the door jamb at about shoulder height. Round your back and lean back, holding on to the doorway. Hold the stretch for 10 to 60 seconds.

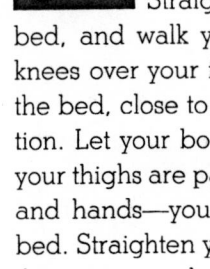 **Pump the Bed.** Sit on the edge of the side of a sturdy bed, your hands on the edge of the bed on both sides of you, knuckles away from the bed. Straighten your arms so that your buttocks lift off the bed, and walk your feet away from the bed. Now align your knees over your feet—your buttocks are now slightly forward of the bed, close to it but not touching it. This is your starting position. Let your body weight down by bending your elbows until your thighs are parallel to the floor. All your weight is on your feet and hands—your body is "sitting" in the air, not touching the bed. Straighten your arms to raise yourself up—do not "help" by thrusting your hips or using your legs. Alternate bending your elbows and straightening your arms, lowering and raising your body. Your triceps (back of the upper arms) are doing the work. Make this more difficult by walking your feet out farther away from the bed (intermediate level) or prop your feet on a sturdy chair (advanced level) so your body is completely suspended.

Sit on the Wall. The phantom chair is a great quadriceps (front of thigh) strengthener: Stand with your back against a wall, and slowly slide down, walking your feet away from the wall so they stay right under your knees, until your thighs are taking your weight and you look like you're sitting on an invisible chair. Hold that pose until your thighs tell you to get up.

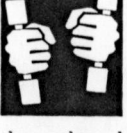

Advanced Phantom Chair. If Sit on the Wall is too easy, try this once you've gotten into position: Lift one leg and put the heel on the other knee. Leave it there. The next day, do this exercise on the other leg.

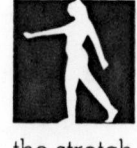

Doorway Chest Stretch. Stand in a doorway, hands gripping the door jamb at about shoulder height. Walk through the doorway, still holding on, until you feel a nice stretch in the chest and shoulders. Hold the stretch for 10 to 60 seconds.

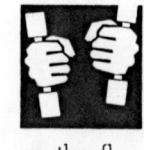

Push the Bed. Do push-ups against your bed, with your feet on the floor, hands on the bed. Be careful not to let your body sag. Advanced: Do push-ups with your feet on the bed (shoes off!) and your hands on the floor.

Push the Stairs. If push-ups against your bed are too easy but full push-ups on the floor are too hard, do your push-ups with your hands a couple of steps up from your feet. The higher your upper body is compared to your feet, the easier the push-ups. Likewise, the higher your feet are compared to your upper body, the harder the push-ups.

You Got Rhythm

If you like push-ups—or the change in muscle tone you see when you do them regularly—spice up your routine with rhythm variations like these. Be careful to keep good form and not let your belly dip.

1. **3 and 3:** Let yourself down for 3 seconds, push up for 3 seconds. Do 2 repetitions.
2. **2 and 4:** Let yourself down for 2 seconds, push up for 4 seconds. Do 2 repetitions.
3. **4 and 2:** Let yourself down for 4 seconds, push up for 2 seconds. Do 2 repetitions.
4. **2 and 2:** Let yourself down for 2 seconds, push up for 2 seconds. Do 4 repetitions.

You can also vary your abdominal crunches with similar rhythm changes. Just substitute "curl-up" or "curl-up with a twist" for "push-up" in the above examples.

Curl-Up with a Twist. Lie on your back with your knees bent and feet flat, hands lightly supporting your head or crossed on your chest. As you exhale, contract the abdominal muscles and lift the chest. Then twist slightly at the waist and aim your shoulder (not elbow) toward the opposite knee, continuing to exhale and lift. Inhale returning to center and lowering down. Alternate sides for a total of 16 to 24 repetitions. Try to take a full 8 seconds to complete each repetition: 2 seconds up, 2 seconds twisting, 2 seconds

At Home: Anytime

137

returning to center, and 2 seconds releasing down. These twisting crunches work your obliques, the abdominal muscles that help shape your waist.

Partner Inner/Outer Thigh Press (PG-Rated). Sit on a sturdy chair without armrests, legs together and straight out in front of you. Have your partner stand facing you, legs straddling your legs. Try to open your legs, as your partner resists your motion by trying to hold them closed with his/her thighs. Continue until your thighs are tired or you're laughing too hard to continue, whichever happens first. Switch positions.

Wash the Car. Wash your car using muscle and chamois, not by driving under a spray machine. A 150-pound person burns 102 calories in 30 minutes of washing the car, and you end up with a clean car. In contrast, watching the game on TV in your recliner burns just 34 calories, and then you have to add in the calories from the beer and chips. Though 102 calories might not seem like much, washing your car by hand once a week instead of driving through a car wash adds up to 5,304 calories you wouldn't otherwise burn. That's a body-fat loss of 1½ pounds just by adding a little more activity every week. (Washing walls burns the same calories as washing the car, if that's what you prefer.)

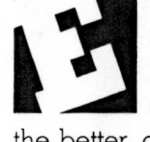 **Side Crunch.** Lie on your back with your knees bent and feet flat, your left hand lightly supporting your head, your right hand extending down your side. Lift your head and chest slightly off the ground, contracting your abdominals. As you exhale, reach your right hand toward your right foot, contracting the right side of your waist. Inhale returning to your starting position. Take 4 seconds per repetition: 2 seconds contracting and 2 seconds releasing. Do 8 to 12 repetitions before switching sides. This exercise works your obliques, the abdominal muscles that help shape your waist.

Wash the Dog. As long as you're thinking cleanliness, how about washing Rover? You'll burn a bit more than 5 calories per minute (159 per half hour), so the bigger the dog (and the less eager for a bath), the better, calorically speaking. See the Resources Appendix to learn exactly how we figured out the calories per minute.

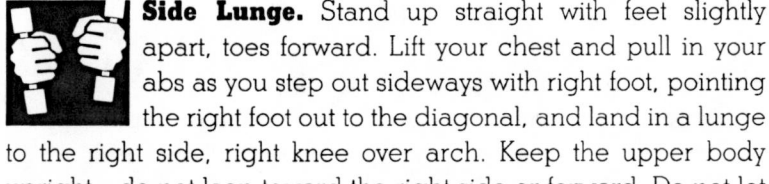 **Side Lunge.** Stand up straight with feet slightly apart, toes forward. Lift your chest and pull in your abs as you step out sideways with right foot, pointing the right foot out to the diagonal, and land in a lunge to the right side, right knee over arch. Keep the upper body upright—do not lean toward the right side or forward. Do not let your knee go past your toes. Push back with your right heel to

return to start. Repeat 8 times before changing sides. You'll strengthen your inner thighs and buttocks as well as your abs and back. Advanced: hold weights at your sides.

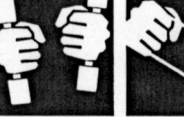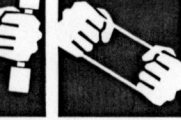 **Dyna-Band At-Home Workout.** Dyna-Bands are stretchy latex resistance bands that work your muscles as though they're lifting weights. They take no space for storage. Here is an exercise routine that strengthens all your major muscle groups. See the additional Dyna-Band exercises in Chapter 5, Chapter 10, and Chapter 16. See the Resources Appendix for more information about Dyna-Bands. You don't need to do all these exercises together, but try to exercise two opposing muscle groups during the same session: chest and back, biceps and triceps, quadriceps and hamstrings. You'll need one band for most exercises; two bands for some. These exercises are done standing unless otherwise noted. If any exercise seems too easy or too difficult, adjust the amount of tension or slack in the band so that the exercise is difficult but not impossible.

- **Push-Ups.** Wrap the band behind your back and get in push-up position (either bent or straight legs, depending on your fitness level), pinning one end of the band under each hand. Adjust the amount of slack in the band to make it snug across your back. Do your regular bent-leg or straight-leg push-ups, keeping the ends of the band anchored under your hands. The added resistance makes the push-ups more difficult. This works your chest, arms, and shoulders.

- **Pull-Down.** Holding the band in both hands, raise your arms high over your head and relax your shoulders down (don't hunch them). Hold your band with your hands about shoulder-width apart. Pull your arms down and out to the side, so you finish with your arms wide open and band touching or almost touching your chest. Slowly return to the starting position. Repeat 8 to 12 times. This works the upper back and shoulders.

- **Seated Leg Press.** Sit on a chair. Raise your right leg, knee bent. Wrap the band around your right foot, holding one end in each hand so that there's tension in the band. Slowly straighten your leg just short of locking your knee. Slowly return to the starting position. Repeat 8 to 12 times before switching sides. This works the quadriceps (front of the thigh).

- **Triceps Extensions.** Hang a small towel around your neck for comfort. Place the band over the towel around the back of the neck, ends hanging in front of your chest. Bend your elbows at right angles and hold the ends of the band. Keeping your elbows close to your body, slowly straighten your arms, keeping your wrists neutral (not crooked). Slowly return to the starting position. Repeat 8 to 12 times before switching sides. This works the back of the upper arms.

- **Biceps Barbell.** Stand with your feet shoulder-width apart, your heels anchoring one end of each of two bands. Hold the other ends in your hands. Wrap the ends over each other, overlapping so you have 6 to 8 inches of double band. This double band is your "barbell." Hold your "barbell" palms up, and perform biceps curls by bending your elbows and bringing the "barbell" toward your shoulder. Keep your elbows at your waist—don't let them ride up—and be careful to keep your back neutral. Slowly return to the starting position. Repeat 8 to 12 times. This works the front of the upper arms.
- **Front Deltoid (Shoulder) Raise.** Hold the middle of the band with your left hand anchored in front of your right hip. Hold one end of the band with your right hand, your right arm down at your side. Lift your right arm in front of your body to shoulder level. Slowly lower. Repeat 8 to 12 times before switching sides. This works the front shoulder muscles.
- **Lateral Deltoid (Shoulder) Raise.** Hold one end of the band with your right hand anchored in front of your left hip. Hold the other end with your left hand, arm slightly bent, keeping your shoulder pressed down. Lift your left arm out to the side to shoulder height. Slowly lower. Repeat 8 to 12 times before switching sides. This works the side shoulder muscles.

- **Rear Deltoid (Shoulder) Press.** Hold the band in front of your chest, one end in each hand. Extend your arms out to the side at shoulder height. Press your arms back. (The range of motion will be small.) Slowly release to starting position. Repeat 8 to 12 times. This works the rear shoulder muscles.
- **External and Internal Rotation.** Stand holding the band with both hands, elbows bent at your waist, your arms extending in front of your body. Pull the band apart by rotating your arms outward, keeping your elbows tucked into your waist. Slowly return to starting position. Repeat 8 to 12 times. This works the rotators, which are small, supportive shoulder muscles that are easily injured when not in shape.

Shoulder Strengthening and Safety Tips

- Lower your shoulders before lifting your arms.
- Keep your back stable—never swing your body into movement.
- Use an easier band for your shoulders than you use for your chest or back.
- Warm up your muscles thoroughly before exercising your shoulders.
- Keep your back in neutral position, neither arched nor rounded.
- Avoid raising your shoulders when raising your arms.
- Lift and lower slowly and with control—do not swing your arms.
- Stretch your shoulders after exercising.

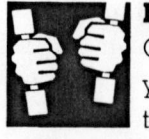 **Bun Busters.** Want to tone and tighten up the rear? Get on the floor on your elbows and knees, keeping your back flat and your abdominals tight. Straighten the right leg out behind you. Now bend the right knee and flex the foot so that the sole pushes toward the ceiling. Press up just a few inches, tightening the buttock and hamstring (back of the thigh) muscles. Control the move as if you were balancing a brick on your foot—don't kick. To work the muscles even harder, press the hipbone down as you push the leg up. Be careful to keep the back from arching. Repeat 8 to 12 times, then switch legs.

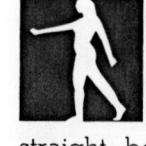 **Doorknob Back Stretch.** To stretch the latissimus dorsi (known in gym circles as "lats"), the large muscles of the back, stand up straight, holding both doorknobs of an open door. Keeping your arms straight, bend your knees to a squat position. Keep your back neutral and lean slightly away from door, stretching the upper lats. Now round your back, stretching the lower lats. Hold 10 to 60 seconds in each position.

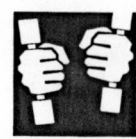 **Bun Buster Variation.** Do the **Bun Busters** above, but add this: After you press up, straighten the leg until it's parallel to the floor, bend it again, and complete the exercise. This makes the hamstrings work harder.

Household Item Workout

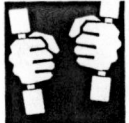 If you wish you had free weights (dumbbells) for strength training but you're not ready to invest in them, you can use common household items to provide resistance. These sample exercises will get you started:

- **Legs with Fanny Pack.** Load a fanny pack or book bag with enough items to make it heavy (how heavy depends on your fitness level). Sit upright in a chair with the strap of the fanny pack over your right ankle. Slowly lift and straighten your right leg, lifting the pack, until your leg is parallel to the floor. Tighten your quadriceps (front of thigh), hold for 4 seconds, and release. Repeat 8 to 12 times, then switch legs. Be careful to keep sitting upright—avoid collapsing forward.
- **Biceps with Bag.** Fill an extra-strength grocery bag with 5 to 8 pounds of canned food. Stand holding the weighted grocery bag in your right hand, palm up. Keeping the elbow firmly against your waist, bend your arm, bringing the bag-holding hand toward your shoulder. Slowly release. Repeat 8 to 12 times, then switch arms. This strengthens the biceps, the front of the upper arms. Be careful to keep your wrist and forearm in line—avoid bending your wrist.
- **Squats with Bags.** Fill two extra-strength grocery bags with 5 to 8 pounds of canned food each. Stand up straight, holding the bags at your sides. Keeping your back neutral (neither arched nor rounded), bend your legs and sit back, as if you were going to sit in a chair a ways behind you. Your knees should stay right above your toes, not forward of them. Squat down until you're almost in a seated position (without a chair, of course), then straighten up. Repeat 8 to 12 times.

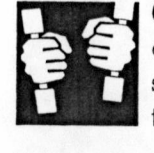 **Chair Squats.** Hover over a chair as if you were going to sit in it. Sit almost all the way down, then straighten up again as if you changed your mind. Do this 8 to 12 times, working the thighs and buttocks.

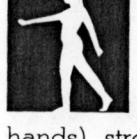 **Chest and Shoulder Stretch.** Sit on the floor in a comfortable position. Roll your shoulders back and clasp your hands behind your body. Push your arms back (as if someone behind you were pulling your hands), stretching your chest and shoulders. Keep your shoulders relaxed and lowered.

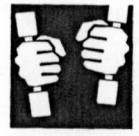 **Stair Calf Raises.** Stand on the stairs with the balls of your feet on the step, letting your heels drop down. Exhale, pushing up on the balls of your feet. Hold for 4 seconds, then slowly lower to starting position. Rise straight up—avoid leaning forward. Repeat 8 to 12 times, then switch legs. This works your abdominals as well as your legs if you don't hold on to the wall or railing.

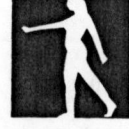 **Neck Stretch.** Sit on the floor in a comfortable position. Hold your right wrist behind your waist with your left hand and pull gently down, relaxing your shoulder. At same time, let your head drop toward your left shoulder, stretching your neck. Change sides.

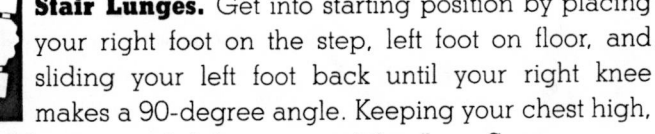

Stair Lunges. Get into starting position by placing your right foot on the step, left foot on floor, and sliding your left foot back until your right knee makes a 90-degree angle. Keeping your chest high, bend and lower your left knee toward the floor. Squeeze your buttocks and straighten up. Repeat 8 to 12 times, then switch legs. Keep your front knee over the arch—do not let your knee go forward of your toes.

Floor Stretching Tips

When your muscles are tight from exercise, stress, illness, or a long day's work, the easiest way to relax them is to lie down on the rug and stretch. Stretching lengthens contracted muscles, lets them release tension, and relaxes your whole body and mind, as well as maintaining or increasing flexibility. Stretching at the end of the day also readies you for sleep. Floor stretches are especially relaxing because you don't have to worry about balancing or holding on to anything.

- Breathe deeply and slowly, exhaling through the mouth as you sink more deeply into the stretch.
- Relax your whole body into the stretch.
- Stretch to your comfortable limit without forcing.
- Relax into each stretch for 10 to 60 seconds.
- Never bounce or force a stretch.

At Home: Anytime

147

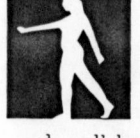 **Quadriceps Stretch.** Lie on your right side. Rest your head on your right arm. Bend your left leg, keeping your shoulder, hip, and knee in a line. Hold your left foot with your left hand behind your body and pull back comfortably, stretching the front of the thigh and hip. Change sides. For more intense stretch, press your hips forward as you pull your foot back. Do this stretch after any aerobic exercise and after squats and lunges.

Leg Stretch. Lie on your back on the floor, both legs bent and feet flat. Bring your right leg in toward your chest and hold the back of the thigh with both hands. Extend your right leg up, foot toward the ceiling, straightening to the point of comfort. Alternate slowly pointing and flexing the right foot, stretching your calf and shin. Repeat 5 times, then switch legs. Do this stretch after any aerobic exercise.

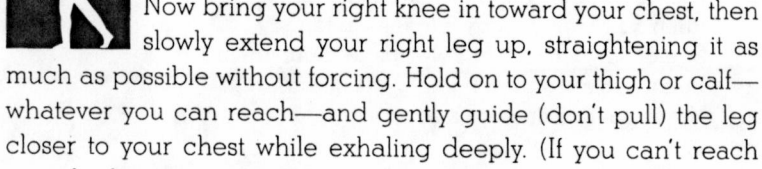 **Hamstring Stretch.** Lie on the floor on your back with your knees bent, feet flat, back pressing down. Now bring your right knee in toward your chest, then slowly extend your right leg up, straightening it as much as possible without forcing. Hold on to your thigh or calf—whatever you can reach—and gently guide (don't pull) the leg closer to your chest while exhaling deeply. (If you can't reach your thigh, wrap a towel around it and hold on to the ends of the

towel.) When you reach your limit, bend your knee slightly, then straighten your leg again; the muscle will probably relax into the stretch a little more. Then bend the knee, lower your leg, and stretch the other side.

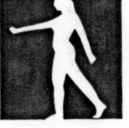 **Buttock Stretch.** Lie on your back on the floor, both legs bent and feet flat. Put your right heel or calf on your left knee. Bring up your left leg toward your chest. Hold your left thigh with both hands and pull it in toward your chest, stretching your buttocks and outer thigh. (If you can't reach your thigh, wrap a towel around it and hold on to the ends of the towel.) Repeat with other leg. Relax your neck and back—don't arch.

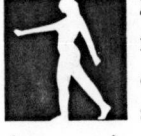 **Back Stretch.** Get on your hands and knees on the floor. Let your buttocks sink back toward your heels as you stretch your arms forward, lengthening your spine. Relax, stretching back. If you wish to intensify the stretch, walk your fingers forward away from your body.

At Home: Anytime

149

12

Chapter 12

9 **Social Shape-Ups** 3

6

ONE OF THE BEST WAYS TO KEEP AN ACTIVE LIFESTYLE interesting and enjoyable is to integrate physical activities into your social life. Get together with friends to enjoy energetic activities together. Consider leisure pursuits that give you the opportunity to talk to friends as you keep moving. Make recreational plans with other active people you meet, expanding your circle of friends and helping each other stay on track. Choose someone's favorite activity, something you all enjoy, or something brand new that just might be fun. The health benefits of physical activity will be a fringe benefit—the best part is that you'll enjoy each other's company and have a good time together. By enjoying active, social activities in the evening and on the weekend, you'll get plenty of extra exercise, and you'll enjoy yourself and your companions.

Fling Your Feet. What kind of social life can you have keeping your sofa warm watching TV? Go dancing. Pick a hot spot where dancing wins over drinking. Don't know how to dance? You'll find dance lessons of all types—ballroom, square, swing, and line dancing, to give just a few examples—at local dance clubs and community centers. Depending on tempo, type, and intensity, 1 hour of social dancing burns 200 to 375 calories (see "Dance Away Calories," following). Compare this to 1 hour of staying home and watching TV, which burns only 68 calories. Plus, when you're home, you're likely to scarf down snacks, which could add several hundred calories during each sitcom to the fat storage on your thighs or belly.

Belly Up to the Barre. Maybe social dancing isn't your thing, but you've always wanted to tap dance or learn ballet, or belly dancing, or flamenco, or hip-hop. Enroll in a class this week. You'll get your aerobic exercise, become stronger and more flexible and coordinated, and discover new ways to enjoy movement. Please don't scoff at this because you think you're too old—it's never to late to discover the joy of dance, and you'll find local classes that warmly welcome mature students.

Dance Away Calories

How many calories can you burn dancing? It depends on the intensity and speed of your movement. Here are some examples of how many calories a 150-pound person burns doing 1 hour of each of these kinds of dancing, according to *Medicine and Science in Sports and Exercise* from the American College of Sports Medicine. And keep in mind that an evening of social dancing might keep your feet moving for a couple of hours or more, so you might burn twice this many calories in an evening.

- Very fast ballroom, traditional American Indian: 375
- Ballet, modern, twist, jazz, tap, jitterbug: 327
- Fast ballroom, disco, folk, square, line dancing, Irish step, polka, contra, country, Greek, Middle Eastern, hula, flamenco, belly, swing: 306
- Slow ballroom: waltz, foxtrot, samba, tango, mambo, cha-cha: 204

Martial Your Forces. Enroll in a martial arts class, then practice your moves evenings when you don't have class. You'll learn to calm down and focus—useful skills for the rest of your day—and might learn skills that can save your life. Originally, all the martial arts were fighting forms, as the name implies. Over the centuries, some—such as tai chi—have evolved into gentle, graceful exercise traditions that seem removed from their roots in fighting. Others remain combat forms and are taught as self-defense. There are many different martial arts, and within each there are many different approaches. Most teach you strength, balance, flexibility, and mental focus.

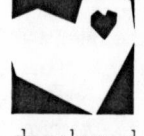

Get in Line. You say you'd like to dance but you don't have a partner or your partner isn't interested? Don't let that stop you! Line dancing, originally exclusive to country/western dance, has developed into a popular recreational dance form that spans all ages and types of music, and you don't need a partner. You're likely to find teens as well as their grandparents boot-scooting, lock-stepping, and hip-bumping their way across the floor. Line dancers dance in rows and learn specific choreography to a particular dance. At a certain point, they all turn and face another direction and start the dance again. A particular line dance might flow to a slow cha-cha beat or tear up the floor at warp speed. Some of the thousands of line dances are simple enough for a two-left-footed first-timer to pick up easily, others are complex enough to tax the brains of the most experienced dancers, and most are in the middle. Many people who never considered themselves dancers get hooked on line dancing—try it!

Walk Your Talk. Plan an outing to a museum, zoo, historic park, botanical gardens, or theme park with a friend, a date, or the family. You'll have plenty of time for conversation as you enjoy the place you're visiting and the good company, and you'll hardly notice how much you're walking. Wear comfortable shoes!

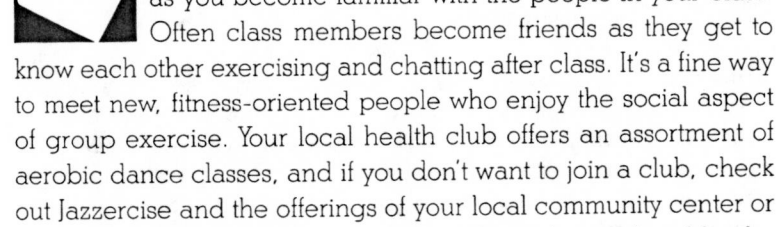 **Aerobic Dance.** Yes, aerobic dance is great exercise—it's designed to be. It's also a good social activity as you become familiar with the people in your class. Often class members become friends as they get to know each other exercising and chatting after class. It's a fine way to meet new, fitness-oriented people who enjoy the social aspect of group exercise. Your local health club offers an assortment of aerobic dance classes, and if you don't want to join a club, check out Jazzercise and the offerings of your local community center or parks and recreation department. In case you're confused by the class descriptions, here's what the nomenclature means:

- **High impact:** This is the original, high-intensity aerobic dance, full of jumps, jogs, kicks, and jacks. "High impact" means that there's jumping involved. This form of aerobic dance burns the most calories and is great for the under-40 set, but might be hard on older joints. A 150-pound person burns 238 calories in 30 minutes.
- **Low impact:** No jumping here, so low impact is kinder on your joints. A 150-pound person burns 170 calories in 30 minutes of an average low-impact aerobics class, although the instructor can make the intensity lighter or stronger.
- **"Hi-lo" or mixed impact:** This class combines some low-impact moves with some high-impact moves, so you get intervals of lower and higher intensity.

Single and having trouble finding companions for outdoor activities? Wish you knew where to meet people who like to hike, bicycle, or camp? Join a singles outdoor activity group. Many regions have local singles activities groups. Do a Web search, or see your local paper for their events. Or you could explore a national group like Sierra Singles (*www.sierraclub.org/singles/index.asp*) or a group with your religious affiliation. Combining exercise with keeping an eye open for Mr./Ms. Right at least ensures that you get your exercise, and it's far healthier than hanging out in bars (where you won't meet that Special Person anyway) and much more enjoyable than answering personal ads. Plus, if you do meet someone you want to date, you already know that he or she is an active person, too.

Pedal Play. Take a bicycle ride with a date or friends, and explore nearby country roads. Your local bike shop has books and maps of good rides with minimal traffic and can advise you about the best places to stop for rest and lunch. Cycling is a heavy calorie burner if you include hills and bike fast; but even if you go at a leisurely pace on a flat road and stop to look at the scenery, you'll have a great time and get plenty of exercise. Calories burned by a 150-pound person in 1 hour of cycling range from 172 (leisurely pace, less than 10 miles per hour) to 681 (vigorous effort, 14 to 15.9 miles per hour).

Take a Date Hike. A date doesn't have to be a movie or dinner. Plan a hike and a picnic lunch at a romantic spot at the coast or in the woods. Besides exercise, you'll enjoy getting into nature, slowing down your frantic pace, and getting a chance to talk to your date and get to know him or her better. Advanced: Carry all the gear yourself.

Play Tourist. You don't have to go far or spend a lot of money to get out of town and become a tourist. Figure out how far away from home you can get in a couple of hours or less, and take a day trip with a friend or honey, exploring a new area (or an area you love and don't visit very often) on foot. Wander in town, in the countryside, whatever strikes your fancy. Be sure to wear comfortable shoes, because even at a slow pace, your tootsies are bound to feel the effects of a day's sightseeing. If you live in a large city, you don't even have to leave town—just choose a part of the city you're not familiar with and wander around.

Play Tennis Badly. Would you believe that the worse you play tennis, the more calories you burn? It's the running and lunging that burn the calories, not hitting the ball, and the more you have to chase the ball, the better for your body (although not for your game).

So get out on the court and play doubles with friends, and laugh your way through lots of missed balls. You'll also condition your legs, thighs, shoulders, and upper arms.

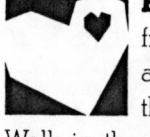 **Beach Games.** A day at the beach with family or friends gives you plenty of opportunity for physical activity. Run on the sand, which burns more calories than running on the road and is much more fun. Walk in the sand, which massages your feet, strengthens your toes, and helps to condition your feet. Play Frisbee, catch, or beach volleyball. Don't forget the sun block!

Get Wet

Forget an air-conditioned movie on a sweltering Saturday afternoon. Instead, head for the pool, lake, or river, and cool off in the water while you burn calories. How many? The following list shows how many calories a 150-pound person burns in 30 minutes of these activities. (Compare this with burning just 34 calories in a half hour of movie-watching, usually accompanied by a large, movie-theater popcorn with butter contributing 1,640 calories and almost 4 days' allotment of saturated fat to your waistline!)

- Canoeing, rowing: 102 to 238, depending on speed and effort
- Diving, body surfing, board surfing, water volleyball: 102
- Treading water: 136 to 341, depending on effort
- Water aerobics, water calisthenics: 136

- Kayaking: 170
- Water skiing, leisurely swimming: 204
- Scuba diving, swimming backstroke: 238
- Swimming laps: 238 to 341, depending on speed and effort
- Swimming breaststroke: 341

Tee Off. You can play golf and barely exert yourself, or you can forgo the cart and get some real exercise. A 150-pound person playing golf for 1 hour burns 306 calories walking and carrying clubs and 238 using a power cart. If miniature golf is more your speed—or if you'd like an activity to do with your children—you'll still burn 204 calories per hour.

Partner Stretches. Stretching doesn't have to be a solitary activity. Stretching with a partner is an enjoyable and beneficial way to increase your flexibility. Partner stretching lets you stretch more deeply than you can by yourself and safely increase your limits of flexibility. You'll find that you can stretch areas and muscle groups that are difficult or impossible to reach on your own. Here are some sample partner stretches—you're bound to discover more.

- **Straight-Legged Pull:** Sit on the floor facing your partner. Both of you have your legs closed and straight in front, with your feet against your partner's feet. Each of you holds one end of a towel. (If you're both quite flexible, you can hold hands without a towel.) One partner leans back slowly, gently pulling the other partner forward. Reverse. This stretches the upper and middle back, shoulders, arms, and hamstrings (back of thighs).

- **Lower Back Stretch:** The stretching partner lies on his or her back on a bench or table, knees bent, feet in the air. The assisting partner puts one hand on the back of the stretching partner's thighs near the knee, the other under the feet, and presses the legs toward the chest gently. Switch roles.
- **Open-Legged Press:** Sit on the floor facing away from your partner, legs apart. Your partner kneels behind you, pressing his or her hands gently against the middle of your back. Let your upper body drop forward very slowly to your personal comfort. Switch roles. This stretches the lower back and inner thighs.
- **Chest and Shoulder Release:** Sit on a low-backed chair or bench, hands behind your neck. Your partner stands behind you, holding your elbows and gently pulling back as you exhale. Stay relaxed and passive, letting go of tension and sinking into the stretch. This chest and shoulder stretch feels particularly good after a day of desk work.

Partner Stretching Tips

Stretching with a partner carries more responsibilities than stretching on your own. Follow these guidelines to keep your partner stretches safe, effective, comfortable, and enjoyable:

- Communicate clearly with your partner, making sure the other person understands your limits and you understand your partner's.
- Breathe deeply, not only to relax into the stretch, but also to communicate with your partner.
- When the stretching person exhales, the assisting partner exerts gentle pressure.
- Always push or pull gently and slowly. Never bounce or force a stretch.
- If you're the assisting partner, tell your stretching partner when you're ready to release the stretch. Then release very slowly—don't let go abruptly.

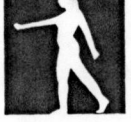 **Leave Your Seat.** If you're attending a play or concert, get away from your seat during intermission to shake out your legs and stretch your back and neck. Even better, take a brisk walk outside for 5 minutes, then return and stretch your back and neck while you're waiting to get back to your seat. Even a 5-minute venture outside will leave you refreshed and eager for Act 2. The following stretches won't attract much attention.

- **Neck Stretch.** Let your head drop to the right side, reaching your left arm down toward the floor. For a more intense stretch, gently pull your head down with your right hand. Hold 10 seconds or more. Release your right hand and let your head roll slowly forward, then slowly to the left side. Repeat the stretch on that side.
- **Back Stretch.** Clasp your hands, turn them palms outward, and reach your arms as far in front of you as you can, rounding your back. Hold 10 seconds or more. Then, in the same position, slightly lift one side and hold, then the other.

12

Chapter 13

9 # Getting
It Together:
Equipping Yourself 3

6

YOU DON'T HAVE TO SPEND MUCH MONEY—or any at all, if you'd rather not—in order to do the exercises in this book. With the right shoes, comfortable clothing, and perhaps a strength-training tool like resistance bands, you can do everything in this book. But you may be wondering whether you'd burn calories faster or slim your thighs thinner with the right gadget, as they promise on television. Here's the skinny.

Choose Your Shoes

The right shoes can make all the difference. Walking shoes are best for walking, running shoes for running, and so on. If you do a variety of activities, a cross-training shoe is probably fine, but if you concentrate on one activity three or more times a week, buy shoes that are designed for that activity. They will keep you most comfortable, help you perform better, and protect you against injuries. Likewise, choose a shoe that fits the unique features of your feet properly, not just your activity. Look for these features for your activity and for your feet:

- **Walking:** Extra shock absorption at the heel, "rocker" soles that let you roll through the foot, smooth tread.
- **Running, aerobic dance:** Enough cushioning to absorb impact, heel stability, soft upper, lightness, good traction.
- **Court sports:** Thinner sole for ankle stability during side-to-side movements. It's best to choose a shoe specific to your court sport, such as tennis, basketball, or volleyball.
- **High arch:** Extra cushioning.
- **Flat feet:** More motion control.
- **Bunions:** Wide toe box.
- **Arch pain:** Arch support.
- **Ankle weakness:** High-tops with ankle support.

You'll get the biggest selection at a specialty athletic-shoe store. Usually the salespeople know athletic shoes well—how they should fit, which shoes are best for which activity, and so on. That's not true in a department or discount store.

Fit Your Feet

When you're buying athletic shoes, follow these guidelines from the American Orthopaedic Foot and Ankle Society (*www.aofas.org/athletic shoes.asp*) for getting the right fit:

- Try on shoes at the end of the day or after exercising, when your feet are largest.
- Wear the same socks that you'll wear when you exercise in these shoes.
- Make sure the shoe grips your heel firmly.
- Be sure you can freely wiggle all of your toes when the shoe is on your foot. There should be at least one thumb's width of space from the longest toe to the end of the toe box.
- Choose shoes that feel comfortable as soon as you try them on. You shouldn't need to break them in.
- Walk or run a few steps in your shoes. They should be comfortable.

Cotton Clothing Cautions

Yes, cotton is a natural fiber, and exercise is a natural activity, but the two don't necessary go best together. Cotton, wonderful as it is, holds moisture and gets soggy. It's fine for stretching and other non-sweaty activities, but for aerobic exercise, you'll be more comfortable in the new synthetic fibers (you'll see them in workout wear by all the major companies) that fit without binding and wick moisture away from your body to keep you dry. If you like the feel of cotton, choose a blend of 50 percent cotton and 50 percent synthetic.

No-Bounce Bra

Do you need a sports bra? If you have large breasts or if your activity makes your breasts bounce, a sports bra will keep you more comfortable. Fortunately, we've come a long way since the days when sports bras bound and flattened your chest (whatever its original size and shape) so you looked like a twelve-year-old boy, and you couldn't wait to get out of them. Now you have many choices, styles, sizes, and features to choose from, and some are comfortable enough to wear all day.

There are two basic types of sports bras:

- **Encapsulation:** This shapes you with molded cups, looking more like a normal bra, but with firmer support. You'll have curves under your clothes. Large-breasted women will find this type more comfortable than compression bras.
- **Compression:** This bra flattens your breasts against your body (but more comfortably than the original sports bras) and prevents movement.

Buy a bra that fits firmly enough to control breast bouncing or any breast movement that could lead to chafing, without interfering with breathing. Be sure you get enough support, especially if you're large-breasted. Make sure the seams don't pinch and the straps don't slip. Try doing jumping jacks in the dressing room to test the bra's support, fit, and comfort during physical activity.

Briefly Speaking

What about underwear? Both genders need nonbinding under-wear that doesn't trap moisture or have seams in unseemly places. Men often choose compression shorts—tight-fitting, stretchy shorts made of nylon and spandex—instead of a jockstrap for many sports and activities. They stretch and breathe better than ordinary cotton briefs. If you're not going to get super sweaty, briefs of a 50 percent cotton and 50 percent synthetic blend will be fine.

Buying Home Equipment

If you like working out on cardio machines, such as a treadmill, stair climber, rower, or ski machine, you might find it a pleasure and a timesaver to have your own machine at home. Buying your own quality cardio equipment is a financial investment, but it pays off in time and convenience. A home machine insures that you have no wait, no driving, no scheduling, no hassles—and you can hop on it for a quick fitness break whenever you want. Depending on where the machine is set up, you can watch the news or supervise the kids while you're working out.

Today's technology offers you a biomechanically engineered piece of equipment built to last; the better models perform amazing feats. Whether you're biking, running, walking, or step-ping, most cardio machines have built-in programs so you can do hills and intervals or stay at a fat-burning pace. Some machines come equipped with a wireless chest-strap heart monitor, which reads your heart rate and adapts your workout to keep you in your target range, easing up when your heart rate goes too high and adding speed or incline if you're too low. Some let you create customized programs, with exactly the speed, intensity, variety, and resistance that you want. A few do everything but sing to you and wash your socks.

These bells and whistles may make the difference between a workout that is terminally bor-r-r-ring and one that motivates you to come back day after day, but they'll also raise the price. If they'll get you to stick with your workout program, they're worth the extra expense. But if you don't care about these features, you'll pay far less for comparable equipment.

While you don't have to buy top of the line, do shop at exercise-equipment specialty stores. You won't be happy or motivated with the cheap machines you'll find in sporting goods or department stores. They're flimsy, noisy, and uncomfortable. The salespeople are not trained about the nuances or even the bare essentials of the equipment; often they don't have the vaguest idea what a good machine looks, feels, or sounds like or what's inside.

Exercise-equipment specialty stores, on the other hand, have knowledgeable salespeople who make it their business to know the machines inside and out. They can help you choose a machine that will please you and keep you exercising.

Do not order an exercise machine from a television ad

unless you can try out that exact brand and model in person!

The bottom line: Don't buy it before you try it. Go to the store wearing exercise clothes, allow plenty of time, carry a towel and water bottle, and become your own personal tester at the equipment store. Ultimately, you are the judge of which machine fits you, suits you, works you out the way you like, and motivates you to hop on and keep going.

Cardio Checklist

Take this checklist with you when you shop for cardio equipment.

1. **Fit:** Is this machine appropriate for your size and stride or stroke?
2. **Feel:** Does the equipment feel sturdy and steady? Is the motion smooth, rhythmic, and reasonably quiet?
3. **Intensity:** Can you go fast enough and hard enough for your fitness level? Can you get your heart rate into target range and keep it there?
4. **Motivation:** Do you genuinely enjoy this type of equipment? Does it have the quality and options that will inspire you to work out on it time after time?
5. **Console:** Is the monitor display easy to read? Does it give you useful information? If the machine is programmable, how difficult is that to learn?
6. **Service:** What home maintenance is required? In case of a problem, can the machine be serviced locally?
7. **Warranty:** Look for a warranty that covers two to three years for parts and at least one year for labor.

Save Your Money

Many exercise machines or gadgets don't do much, and they especially don't do what they're supposed to do. Many others allow you to do what you could do perfectly well without them. In general, any item that claims it "spot reduces" is pulling your leg, because spot reducing is a myth. You can't "burn" fat from any one, designated part of the body, unfortunately. The sad rule of thumb (or, more accurately, rule of thigh, hip, or belly) is that the last place you gained weight is the first place you'll lose it, and the last place you'll lose it is the first place you gained it. Who said life was fair? It's genetics—your body is programmed to store fat in certain areas. No number of workouts with the thigh machine will change that.

Here are some machines you don't need:

- **Ab rollers:** These late-night television hot sellers promise you perfect crunches. Well, gee—you can do perfect crunches just as well on your own, following the instructions for **The Perfect Crunch** in Chapter 10. You don't need any machine or gadget to work your abdominals effectively. We're suckers for ab doodads because we want a quick shortcut to a flat midriff. But the abdominals are muscles like any others, and they respond to the correct training—nothing mysterious about that. Realize, though, that you can do crunches or use the latest ab machine until the cows come home, and if you have body fat covering your middle, your abdominal muscles won't show. So the key to abdominal definition is not only working your abs, but cutting calories and doing enough regular, calorie-burning exercise to lose the extra weight. Just working the abs does not "burn" belly fat. But exercises targeting the abdominals will strengthen them and—this is really good news—help strengthen your back. Ab rollers actually limit the muscles you use and the variety of abdominal exercises you can do. Bottom line: Learn good form and do it on your own.

- **Thigh machines:** These best-selling pieces of plastic promise the inner thighs of a star. There's no way you can use a gizmo to work one part of the body and expect to lose fat in that area. There's no such thing as spot reducing! (Have we repeated this enough?) These machines provide resistance for strengthening this area, but they're expensive (you're paying for that late-night advertising, after all) and no better than super-inexpensive resistance bands (see Dyna-Bands in the Resources Appendix).
- **Aerobic rider:** You might be tempted to pick one up cheap at a garage sale. Despite the inflated calorie-burning claims, these riders only deliver if you're an absolute beginner. Aerobic-rider exercisers, even using the machine correctly, burn only 50 percent or fewer calories than they would burn walking on a treadmill. And despite the full-body workout

claims, the only muscles consistently exercised on all brands were the hamstrings.

- **The latest gizmo:** We're sure that by the time this book comes out, there will be some new machine or doodad guaranteed to do something magical to your stubborn fat stores and get you in shape with no effort at all. Remember the premise of this book—you don't have to do intense, vigorous exercise to reap the health and weight-loss benefits, but you *do* have to move a lot. Use common sense and ask yourself whether you need this gadget to increase the physical activity in your everyday life or whether you can do the same thing with less-expensive equipment or no equipment. The answer to the first question is usually "No"; the answer to the second is usually "Yes!"

Beware, Be Wary

It's late at night, and you're ver-r-r-ry sleepy. Your eyelids flutter, and you know you should go to bed, but your remote has fallen between the sofa cushions and you find yourself riveted to the Fitness Infomercial That Will Change Your Life. Somehow your charge card materializes in one hand and your phone in the other, and you're dialing.

Wake up!

Whew, you saved yourself this time, but how many times have you embarrassed yourself by ordering a fitness gimmick or diet aid that's ineffective or useless and used it seldom, if at all? Do you throw a blanket over the pile of late-night television exercise gizmos stuffed at the back of your closet? If you're like the typical consumer, you use an infomercial purchase four times before dumping or hiding it.

Now we're not branding all products advertised on television as rip-offs. Some of these products are very good. Many are not. The point is that people are swayed to buy not by evidence of quality, but by shrewd sales promises, language tricks, and innuendoes. Don't call yourself stupid or gullible. These advertisers are slick. Educate yourself before you buy. And make sure you're wide awake and well informed before you whip out your credit card. (Learn more about how to recognize quackery by reading "Quack Alert" at *www.joan price.com/articles/quack.htm.*)

So What Do You Really Need?

Depending on which activities you enjoy and what motivates you to stick with them, you might need nothing more than comfortable clothing and the right shoes (see above). There are a few pieces of equipment that might enhance your exercise experience:

- **Pedometer:** If your main activity is walking, a pedometer that either counts steps or records the miles you cover can help you stay on track. (See the Resources Appendix for more information.)
- **Resistance bands:** If you'd like an inexpensive, easy alternative to lifting weights for strengthening your muscles, resistance bands like Dyna-Bands are super tools. (See the Resources Appendix for more information.)

- **Outdoor bicycle:** If you live in an area that's safe for cycling, without much traffic, a bicycle might be just the ticket to getting outside and enjoying aerobic exercise.
- **Exercise videos:** If you enjoy exercising indoors, following a leader, and working out to music, exercise videos will give you an instant and private exercise class. (See Chapter 9 to learn how to choose and use an exercise video.)

12

Chapter 14

9   **Kid Stuff:**   3
Family Fitness

6

I N 1999, 13 PERCENT OF CHILDREN aged 6 to 11 and 14 percent of adolescents aged 12 to 19 in the United States were overweight, according to *The Surgeon General's Call to Action to Prevent and Decrease Overweight and Obesity*. The number of overweight teens has nearly tripled over the past two decades. Overweight children are more likely to be at risk for heart disease, type 2 diabetes, high blood pressure, and some forms of cancer. Overweight adolescents have a 70 percent chance of becoming overweight or obese adults—80 percent if they have an overweight parent. They also face peer discrimination, often **175** leading to poor self-esteem and depression. Although genetics certainly play a role, the main causes are lack of physical activity and poor eating habits. With children choosing television, computers, and video games over active play, no wonder they're gaining weight.

It's our job to help reverse this trend. Parents have the opportunity to help children stay active and develop into active adults, just by encouraging active play and—very important!—by setting a good example themselves. We can't tell children to "go out and play" when we're parked in front of the television. Better to participate in physical activity *with* our children, to help them find exercise activities that they'll enjoy, and to show them that we're doing exercise activities that *we* enjoy.

Children model behavior they see. If they see an adult enjoying exercise, they'll incorporate physical activity as a positive part of life. If parents are inactive themselves, children are more likely to become sedentary adults. Exercising with children and making this a part of family life is the best way to help children grow up healthy, active, and enthusiastic about movement.

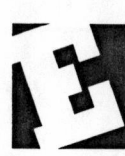 **Tick Tock.** Set time limits for sedentary activities such as video games and television, and use planned physical activities instead of food to reward children's accomplishments.

Walk the Kids. If school isn't prohibitively far away, take the extra time to walk your children to school instead of driving them. This is not only healthier for all of you, but you teach the children (and yourself) to choose walking over riding. Then walk to get them at the end of the day, and walk home a different, more circuitous, route, since you're not racing the late bell on the return trip. You'll get twice the exercise, since you have a round trip each time, and you can go at an aerobic pace returning home in the morning and going to school in the afternoon, when the children aren't with you. If you have a younger child who can't keep up with the others, let the young'un ride a tricycle. (If there's no safe place to store the tricycle at school, you can walk it back home and then to school again in the afternoon for the return trip.)

Child's Choice. Put your school-age child in charge of teaching a new physical activity to the whole family. It might be an active game learned at recess or from another child, a sport, or a recreational activity the child already enjoys. The whole family participates. Another time, a different family member chooses and leads another activity. Who knows, you might learn to skateboard! Make outdoor physical activities an important part of your family fun.

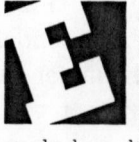**Active Chores.** Make sure your children have household and yard work chores that promote physical activity, like raking leaves, taking out the trash, picking up toys, walking the dog, washing the car, and shoveling snow. Make sure the chore is age-appropriate and never used as punishment.

A Child's Healthy Heart

The American Heart Association (AHA) recommends a daily combination of moderate and vigorous physical activity for both children and adults. Specifically, the AHA suggests the following to help children achieve cardiovascular fitness:

- All children age 5 and older should participate in at least 30 minutes of enjoyable, moderate-intensity activities every day.
- They should also perform at least 30 minutes of vigorous physical activities at least 3 or 4 days each week to achieve and maintain a good level of cardiorespiratory (heart and lung) fitness.
- Children who don't have a full 30-minute activity break each day should have two 15-minute periods or three 10-minute periods in which they can engage in vigorous activities appropriate to their age and stage of physical and emotional development.

Participate in P.E.

Talk to your children's teachers about what they are doing in physical education classes and how you can encourage or supplement these activities. Ask what fitness tests your child will be taking and how you can help your child prepare. Find out how much of the time in each P.E. class children are actually active so that you can make sure your child gets enough additional exercise. Encourage your school to provide physical activities that will lead to lifetime fitness, not just competitive sports.

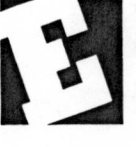 **Get Outdoors.** The outdoors can be a giant playground for the whole family, whatever the age of your child. These outdoor activities will be fun for the family and teach your child the joy of physical activity:

- Go on nature hikes and scavenger hunts
- Rake leaves
- Ride bikes
- Roller skate
- Ice skate
- Fly kites
- Play hide-and-seek
- Play tag
- Have a ball game
- Plant and tend a garden together
- Participate in a park, trail, or coastal cleanup

- Build a snowman
- Play badminton
- Play hopscotch
- Jump rope
- Shoot baskets
- Toss a football
- Play dodge ball
- Climb on the jungle gym
- Play Frisbee
- Play miniature golf
- Play hacky-sack
- Pitch horseshoes

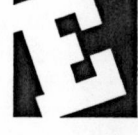 **Lessons for Life.** Enroll your children in classes when they are enthusiastic about learning a sport or active skill, such as swimming, martial arts, gymnastics, horseback riding, or dance.

Standing Rocker. Rocking your baby to sleep feels wonderful to both baby and mom. If you stand while you rock your baby, it will feel the same to the infant, but you'll burn twice as many calories as sitting in the rocking chair. And if you walk around the room holding your baby, you'll burn even more.

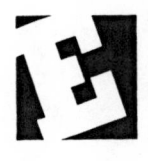

Water Play. The water is an invigorating, playful exercise arena for kids and parents. Whether you have access to a lake, river, or pool, some of these options could be just right for your family:

* Swim
* Play water games
* Learn to dive
* Go kayaking or canoeing
* Pedal a paddleboat
* Go sailing

Mom's Stroller Workout. Take your small child for a walk in the park in a stroller. Walk briskly rather than leisurely. At intervals, stop and do one of these muscle-strengthening exercises, holding on to the stroller handles:

* **Squats:** Bend your knees, keeping your weight back as if you're about to sit in a chair.
* **Outer Thigh Lifts:** Stand on one leg and lift the other leg out to the side slowly.
* **Calf Raises:** Rise onto your toes. Slowly release.
* **Buttock Presses:** Stand on one leg and slightly lift the other leg behind you, pushing your hip forward at the same time.

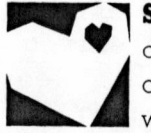 **Soccer Mom.** If your kids play sports, you have to deliver them early before practice or a game, and chances are you just sit around waiting. Instead, walk while you wait. If the school track is free, use it. Otherwise, circle the field or school or park, wherever you happen to be. You'll stay close enough to race back to your spectator spot when it's time, and you'll get your exercise. Encourage other soccer moms to walk with you.

Play, Not Workout

Put the emphasis on play (rather than exercise), recommends the American Heart Association, suggesting these kinds of activities:

- Regular walking, bicycling, and outdoor play.
- Use of playgrounds and gymnasiums.
- Playing with other children.
- Less than 2 hours per day watching television or videotapes.
- Participation in age-appropriate organized sports, lessons, clubs, or sandlot games.
- Daily school or day care physical education, with at least 20 minutes of coordinated large-muscle exercise.
- Opportunities for physical activity that are fun, increase confidence in participating in physical activity, and involve friends and peers.
- Regular family outings that involve walking, cycling, swimming, or other recreational activities.

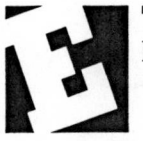 **Tiny Tots Workouts.** Toddlers are naturally active. Encourage this with activities such as these:

* Blow bubbles and chase them.
* Bat balloons to each other.
* Act out animals.
* Dance (unstructured) to your child's favorite music. Add waving and clapping.
* March, jump, and hop together. Add props such as ribbons, scarves, balls, Hula-Hoops, and balloons for variety.
* Let your child dance along when you work out to a grown-up exercise video.

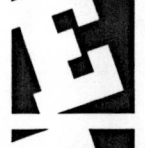 **The Gift That Keeps on Giving.** Buy toys and other gifts that promote physical activity, like balls, active games, and sports equipment.

Active Work. When your child is old enough to seek a part-time or summer job, encourage a job that keeps him or her physically active, such as mowing lawns, delivering newspapers (on foot or bicycle), caddying, or waiting tables.

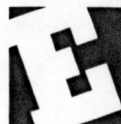 **Borrow a Toddler.** You don't have your own child for stroller or play activities? Or your children would rather play with their friends than with you? Offer to baby-sit a friend's toddler. Your friend will be wild with appreciation for the chance to go for a walk, see a movie, or read a book, and you'll run yourself ragged keeping up with the little tyke. Just don't park the child in front of the television or in the playpen—get outside to the park or play in the yard.

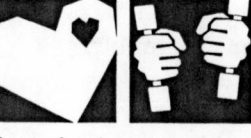 **Teens at the Gym.** Some teenagers blossom when they join a health club. The boys usually gravitate to the weight room, the girls to the aerobics and step classes, though of course the reverse can happen. Both genders enjoy the cardio and weight machines and the social aspect of meeting their friends and making new ones.

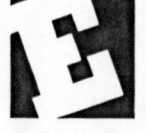 **Track Time.** Go to a local track to get your grown-up exercise, such as brisk walking or jogging. Let the children play on the infield where you can watch them.

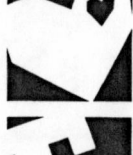 **Walk and Talk.** Those serious family discussions with your older child or teenager don't have to take place in the living room. You can take a walk. You'll cover just as much ground talking and much more walking.

Party Plan. Celebrate a birthday with an activity-oriented party. Invite partygoers to one of these options, and make cake-eating secondary to active fun:

- Hike and picnic
- Backpacking trip
- Day at the beach, with active games
- Kite-flying at the park
- Pool party with swimming and water games
- Ice skating at the local rink
- Skateboarding or rope-jumping games

Teen Dancing. Teenagers of both genders love music and can enjoy dancing, especially if they're introduced to it in a nonpressured, noncompetitive, friendly, enjoyable environment. Your teen might enjoy swing, line dancing, tap, or hip-hop. Some teens who don't like and aren't good at sports will feel comfortable dancing and enjoy it immensely. Since teens are most influenced by their peers, see if your local teen center, community center, or dance studio has dance classes especially for teens. Find out which grown-up dance scenes also welcome teenagers. Look for classes and dance venues where the teenage participants are smiling and having a great time so that your teen sees the experience as fun. Teens who dance are developing a fitness activity that they can continue throughout their adult lives.

========= **Your Overweight Child and Exercise** =========

Do you have an overweight child? *The Surgeon General's Call to Action to Prevent and Decrease Overweight and Obesity* makes these suggestions for parents:

- Let your child know he or she is loved and appreciated whatever his or her weight.
- Focus on your child's health and positive qualities, not your child's weight.
- Be a good role model for your child. If your child sees you enjoying healthy foods and physical activity, he or she is more likely to do the same now and for the rest of his or her life.
- Be physically active yourself, and help your child accumulate 60 minutes or more of moderate physical activity most days of the week.
- Plan family activities that provide everyone with exercise and enjoyment.
- Provide a safe environment for your children and their friends to play actively; encourage swimming, biking, skating, ball sports, and other fun activities.
- Reduce the amount of time you and your family spend in sedentary activities, such as watching television or playing video games. Limit TV time to less than 2 hours a day.

186

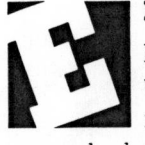 **Musical Calorie Burning.** You wouldn't think that playing a musical instrument is good exercise—and usually you'd be right. But some instruments involve more activity than others. Playing the drums, for example, burns twice as many calories as playing the flute. Ditto for playing any instrument in the marching band.

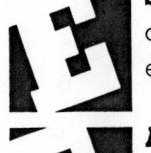 **Send the Kids to Camp.** Summer camp is a wonderful way to keep children physically active and expose them to new activities.

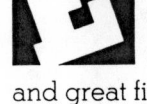 **Adopt a Neighbor.** With the kids, visit an elderly, injured, or very busy neighbor or relative and offer to do some of the outside chores. Mow, rake leaves, shovel snow, or water the garden. It will be family fun and great fitness for your family and a godsend to your neighbor or relative.

=========== **Safety Cautions** ===========

Keep your kids safe as well as fit with these tips:

- Children can safely participate in vigorous sports, but avoid high-contact sports like football and hockey.
- Make sure children have appropriate safety gear for their activities, such as bicycle helmets.

- Avoid activities that involve heavy lifting.
- Children produce more body heat during activity than do adults, so encourage them to drink plenty of water before, during, and after vigorous exercise, especially in warm weather.
- Unfortunately, some people prey on children. Always make sure your children are supervised by an adult when they play outside.

12

Chapter 15

9   Air-Robics   3

6

AIR TRAVEL IS FULL OF STRESS, especially the "hurry-up-and-wait" kind. You can use the waiting time in an airport to de-stress and energize instead of sitting around like a lounge potato, however. Even in the airplane, you can do some stretches and strengtheners. If you choose opportunities to be active in the airport and find ways to move during your flight, you'll arrive feeling healthier and much more energized and relaxed. And the waiting time will go faster!   **189**

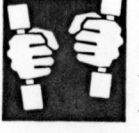 **Lug a Laptop.** If you use a laptop on business travel, carry it in a backpack instead of its case. The weight will be more evenly distributed, and since you're wearing rather than carrying it, shoulder and wrist stress will be minimal. Added benefit: Thieves won't know you're carrying a laptop and will target the guy carrying the snazzy Toshiba case.

 **Terminal Workout.** Instead of sitting around trying to make the newspaper last until boarding time, stash your carryon in a locker and powerwalk the terminal. Walk as fast as possible. If you find any stairs, walk up and down them. You'll have plenty of time to sit *after* you board the plane, so why do more of it than you have to? And you'll feel much better during your flight if you exercise right beforehand. Depending on speed, a 150-pound person will burn this many calories in 30 minutes of walking the terminal (compared to 44 calories sitting and reading the newspaper):

- 2 mph (slow pace): 85
- 3.3 mph (moderate pace): 112
- 3.5 mph (brisk pace): 129
- 4 mph (very brisk pace): 170
- 4.5 mph (very, very brisk pace): 215

Prepare, Phone, and Pack

Before you even leave your house, you can take these steps to make sure your fitness program is your traveling companion.

- **Prepare** by determining which fitness activities you can do in the airport, in a new city, and in a hotel room. Choose activities from this book and others that you really enjoy. Figure out what clothing, gear, and shoes you need to take with you.
- **Phone** the hotel where you will be staying. Ask whether it has a gym or pool or arrangements with a health club nearby, if this appeals to you. Ask about nearby parks, hiking trails, tennis courts, or whatever interests you.
- **Pack** the clothing and lightweight equipment (like a jump rope or Dyna-Bands) you'll need for your activities. Choose clothing that you can wash easily in the sink and that dries quickly, like nylon. Plan to wear your athletic shoes traveling, or pack them in your carryon bag so you can walk the airport. If you have to wear business clothes while traveling, invest in a pair of dress/walking shoes that look like dress shoes but feel like walking shoes. Don't forget sun block for outdoor activities. And, of course, take this book in your carryon!

Move Your Own Body. Avoid the "people movers," those moving belts like flat escalators. You'll spend enough time not moving—don't settle for even more. Instead, walk on your own two feet. If your luggage is heavy, rent a cart and push it—even more exercise!

Luggage Lift. Instead of killing your back dragging your suitcase, strengthen your back by lifting it. While you're waiting in that long line to check your luggage, do bent-over rows: Stand with the left leg forward and bent, resting your left hand on your left thigh, leaning forward from the hip with your back neutral. Grip your suitcase handle with your right hand. Aiming your right elbow toward the ceiling, pull your suitcase straight up until the handle reaches your rib cage. Be careful to keep your back straight and knees bent when you lift—do not round your back or twist when lifting. Slowly release. Do 8 to 12 repetitions before changing sides. (Keep this book handy to show the security people who might express interest in your antics.)

Aisle Aerobics. Too much sitting in a cramped airplane seat feels awful. Worse, it can lead to the rare but potentially deadly travel-related thrombosis—the formation of blood clots, which can, in rare and extreme cases, travel to your heart, lungs, or brain. You've got to get your circulation going while aboard the plane, so get out of your seat and take frequent trips to the restroom and the magazine rack. While you're in the aisle, do a subtle jog (sort of like a bouncing walk) and make the foray last as long as possible.

Flight Food

You can't feel fit if you eat the high-fat, salty, overcooked airline meal. Instead, call your travel agent or airline in advance and ask about special meals. All major airlines offer dietary alternatives for people with special requirements, as long as these meals are ordered in advance. Though airlines vary in their special meal offerings, you can usually order a low-fat or vegetarian alternative. Then once you get on the plane, introduce yourself to the flight attendant as the recipient of the special meal.

Carry your own healthy snacks and bottled water. Even if you're getting a special meal on the flight, the standard waiting time in the airport and the probability of delays might leave you eyeing the calorie-laden pizza in the airport, starving as you sit on the runway, or gobbling the salty, fat-filled nuts once the plane gets in the air. And more airlines are restricting the food they serve on board to cut costs. Nutritious, portable snacks include these:

- Dried fruit
- Trail mix
- Apples
- Bagels
- Low-fat crackers
- Rice cakes
- Carrots
- Dry cereal
- Bananas
- Grapes
- Energy bars
- Pretzels

Air-Robics

193

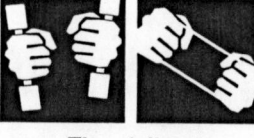 **Band on Board.** Carry a resistance band like a Dyna-Band (see the Resources Appendix) in your carryon, and use it to strengthen a few muscles while in your seat. The following exercises suit a seated position and tight spaces:

- **Chest Strengthener:** Hold the middle of the band with both hands a few inches apart. Cross the hands at the wrist and push toward and past the opposite elbow 8 to 12 times.
- **Biceps Curl:** Hold the middle of the band with both hands close together. Anchor the left hand at the right side of your hip. Keeping your right elbow at your waist, bring the right hand up toward your shoulder, and slowly release it down. Switch sides after 8 to 12 repetitions.
- **Seated Row:** Wrap the middle of the band under your knees. Grip the band with each hand close to where it emerges at your outer thighs. Pull toward your rib cage, squeezing the shoulder blades at the end of the move. This works the large muscles of the back. If you're a small person, you can get more resistance by crossing the ends of the band and holding the left end with the right hand and vice versa.

Ankle Energizer. Sitting in a plane for hours can make your legs and feet swell, look like balloons, and feel like lead. Get out of the seat as often as possible, but when you're stuck under your seat belt, circle your ankles in both directions, and alternate pointing and flexing your feet.

Magazine Drop. You're on the plane, and you'd really like to stretch your back, but you hate to attract attention. Drop the magazine you're reading onto the floor between your feet. Reach for it (be sure your tray is up!) and take your time returning to an upright position.

=========== **Airport Restaurant Tips** ===========

Daniel Sands, M.D., a physician, lecturer, and consultant who travels by air about 25 times a year, looks for these healthful alternatives to the usual airport meal when hunger strikes in an airport:

- **Wraps:** Avoid mayo or fillings like tuna or chicken salad, since they contain mayo.
- **Salads:** Avoid creamy or cheese dressings, like blue cheese and Caesar dressing.
- **Japanese food:** Avoid the fried dumplings called "shu mai" because they are very high in fat. Stick to noodle soups, salads, and (if it looks fresh) sushi.
- **Fruit smoothies:** Aim for fresh fruit rather than canned or frozen.
- **Soup:** Avoid cream soups, cheese soups, or soups containing beef or sausage.

Air-Robics

195

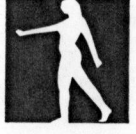 **Light Stretch.** Get a great upper-body stretch from your seat by reaching for the light or air control above you. Take your time adjusting it, pretending that you just can't get it right (should anyone notice). Repeat a few minutes later, reaching with the other arm.

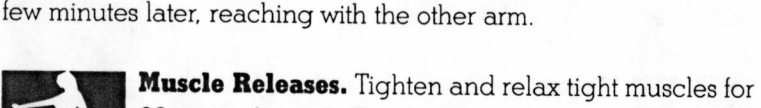 **Muscle Releases.** Tighten and relax tight muscles for 60 seconds each. For example:

- **Thigh:** Extend your leg and contract and release the quadriceps muscles.
- **Abdominals:** Sit up straight and inhale, lifting the rib cage. Exhale into a crunch, contracting the abs.
- **Chest and back:** Wrap your arms around yourself as if you were giving yourself a well-deserved hug. Walk your fingers toward your shoulder blades. Pull your shoulder blades as you curl forward, tightening the chest and stretching the back. Then reverse by rolling your shoulders back, squeezing your elbows together behind you.
- **Face:** Open your face wide—wide eyes, wide jaw—then scrunch it tight. Caution: Only the least inhibited should do this one in public in a well-lighted place! You might want to save this for the bathroom stall.

Of course, if you've got more than 1 minute to spare—and you will, if you're flying—you can keep on tightening and releasing different muscle groups. After 5 minutes, you'll feel like a new person.

============= **1-Minute Stress-Busters** =============

You can do these simple 60-second stress-busters in the airport, in the plane, or anywhere else you need a mental or physical tension-reliever. These easy stress-reducing techniques calm your mind, relax your body, and even bring down your heart rate. Most of these use the mind and leave your body relaxed and motionless, so you won't attract any attention doing them in an airport or plane. Fitness expert and lifestyle coach David Essel, M.S. (*www.davidessel.com*), who travels up to twenty times a year, contributes these tips.

- **Deep Breathing:** Sit still and take 10 deep, slow breaths. Mentally, you'll feel calmer. Physiologically, you'll bring down both your heart rate and your blood pressure.
- **Time Out:** When you find yourself in a stressful situation, count to 10 before you react. The slower you count, the better this works.
- **Mental Vacation:** Close your eyes. Mentally place yourself in an environment that gives you peace and pleasure. Visualize your fantasy place and what you would do there.
- **Body Scanning:** When your body tenses up, close your eyes and do a mental scan of your body, head to toe, to find the areas where your body is reacting to stress. Move that area to increase

blood flow. If your neck is tight, for example, do head circles. If your shoulders are tight, do shoulder shrugs.

- **Lavender Lull:** Pack a small bottle of lavender essential oil, available at all health food stores. Just a whiff of this scent will help your mind and body to become calmer and more peaceful.

12

Chapter 16

9 **Frisky Hotel Workouts** 3

6

HOTEL STAYS AND EXERCISE—they don't seem to go together. But actually, it's easy to incorporate exercise into your travels. When you do, you'll find you're more productive, energetic, and calm, and you'll be able to enjoy your trip and accomplish more. It does take some planning and self-discipline—your routine is disrupted, and it's easy to just let your fitness habit fall by the wayside. Rather than return home wearing extra pounds and having to struggle to get back on track, take your good exercise habit with you. The new city you're visiting and the hotel itself become a playground to explore new exercise options. **199**

Realize first that a session of aerobic exercise—running, brisk walking, dancing, climbing stairs, and other "portable" aerobic exercises—will energize you all day long. Even 5 minutes will invigorate you mentally and physically and decrease stress. Add some simple strengtheners and stretches that take only minutes, and you've got a total program away from home. (For more exercises, see Chapter 3, Chapter 10, and Chapter 11—many of those exercises can be done in a hotel room.)

Concierge Cardio. Ask the concierge at the hotel for the best (most interesting, safest) walking or running route. Often, the concierge will whip out a map for you. At the beginning or end of your day, get outside and see how fast you can cover the route. You'll energize and see new sights. Be sure to carry water and identification, including the name and phone number of your hotel.

Hotel Hotfoot. As soon as you park your bags in your hotel room and inspect the amenities, put your key in your pocket and leave the room. Explore the hotel lobby at a brisk pace. Walk (don't ride) the escalator to the mezzanine and check out the names of the conference rooms (even if you're not attending a conference). Stride to the gym and swimming pool. Walk in and out of the lounge. Walk out the front door and in the side door. By getting your heart rate up right away, even for a few minutes, you release the stress and fatigue of your trip and set your commitment to stay active during your hotel stay.

Explore Aerobically. Take advantage of new scenery and experiences by walking through this new city. See what's around your hotel by walking a few blocks in every direction. If the area around the hotel isn't conducive to walking, drive or take public transportation to an interesting tourist spot, or the old downtown area, or a scenic spot mentioned in the guidebooks, and walk briskly through it, not stopping to shop or eat or meander (don't worry—you can do this later). After you've had your exercise, return to favorite spots that you passed.

Walk to Dinner. Plan a nice dinner at a restaurant a mile or two away from the hotel, and walk to it. Check with your concierge about the best route. Wear athletic shoes and carry dressy shoes for later, if needed. You'll work up an appetite, see more of the city, and not have to regret those extra dinner calories. Be sure to carry water.

Restaurant Rescue

Here's a typical scenario: You end up in a restaurant because (a) someone else chose it; (b) it's close to the hotel; or (c) you're too tired at the end of the day to hassle decision-making. You look at the menu, and there's nothing that supports a healthy lifestyle. Your options are to choose some cream-sauced, calorie-laden, cholesterol-filled belly-bulger—or watch everyone else eat while you pick at a salad.

Yes, you can eat nutritious, low-fat foods when you travel. It takes some planning and self-discipline to avoid the excess fat and salt, but it's worth the bother. If you're used to healthful eating, taking a break from this habit will slow you down and make you feel bloated, sluggish, and uncomfortable. You'll also return home wearing extra pounds. Fortunately, you can create a different reality and take your good nutritional habits with you.

The solution is proactive planning. Long before you're tired and hungry, investigate where you can get healthy meals. Before you leave home, get recommendations from friends, read magazine reviews, and do a Web search for restaurants in that city. Once you get to the new city, peruse the Yellow Pages restaurant ads. Ask the concierge. Then phone the restaurants that end up on your list and make sure they offer foods you like.

If you get stuck in a restaurant of someone else's choice, you can still order proactively. Instead of making your best guess from the menu, say to the waitperson, "I have medical reasons for needing to eat a heart-healthy, low-fat diet. How can you accommodate me?" (You're not lying, even if you haven't seen a doctor in a decade. Who could deny that everyone has medical reasons for eating a heart-healthy diet?) Many restaurants will be happy to prepare something that fits your dietary needs even if it's not on the menu. Just ask before you order.

Hall Hike. Whatever the weather outside, you can hall walk. Just powerwalk the halls of the hotel on your floor, the lobby floor, any old floor, taking the stairs when you want to change floors. Avoid morning and early afternoon, when you're likely to keep bumping into housekeeping carts.

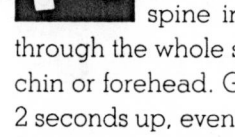

Push-Ups. This is the most effective all-purpose upper-body strengthener. Whether you do push-ups with bent or straight legs, keep your head, neck, and spine in alignment and the abdominals contracted through the whole sequence. Lead with the chest—don't dip the chin or forehead. Go slowly: no faster than 2 seconds down and 2 seconds up, even slower if you're strong. Exhale on the way up. See Chapter 11 for variations on push-ups.

Elevator Avoidance. Skip the elevator and walk to your room. If you're on one of the top floors, take the elevator, but get out three floors below yours and walk from there. If that's too hard at the end of a long day, take the elevator to the floor that is three flights *above* yours, and walk down. Make sure, first, that the door to your floor will open from the stairway—sometimes hotels let you exit but not enter on a guest room floor.

 **Tube Tune-Up.** Channel surf in the morning for exercise programs on television. You can exercise along with the leaders, or use them to motivate you while you do your own workout. If you don't find an exercise program, look for a music channel and dance or do your own exercises to the music.

Travelers' Tips Rescue

Business travelers and public speakers travel as part of their lifestyle. Despite spending a good portion of their life in airports, planes, and hotel rooms, they have to look and feel their best—it's part of the job. These are some of the busiest people you can imagine, yet they manage to motivate themselves to exercise wherever they are. Here's how some of them stay in shape on the road:

- "When I travel, I jog or walk every morning. I like to find a hill to hike up. It reminds me of positive affirmations that program me for climbing other mountains in my business life or relationships."— Thomas (Thom) A. Lisk, LHD, CSE, President/CEO Professional Speakers Bureau Int'l Association, *www.terrificspeakers.com*.

- "I always take running shoes and shorts and do twenty to thirty minutes of aerobics (Jane Fonda style) in my hotel room before breakfast while I watch the news. I developed my routine at home so I don't have to think about it. I also do crunches, push-ups, and lunges for strength training and yoga or stretches before I go to bed or between meetings."—Margaret Moore, President and CEO, Wellcoaches Corporation, *www.wellcoaches.com*.

- "The big issue I have, as a guy who does pretty intense, demanding workouts, is keeping my expectations in check while I'm traveling. The first thing I do is scrap any idea that the workout is going to accomplish a major athletic goal. Instead, I see the workout as playtime for my muscles. Every other part of a business trip is about my company, so the workout is about me. I try out equipment I haven't used before. If I get a chance, I work out with somebody who can teach me something new."—Lou Schuler, C.S.C.S., Fitness Director, *Men's Health*, author of *The Testosterone Advantage Plan* and *The Men's Health Home Workout Bible*.

- "Exercise time on the road is as important as meal time. I walk neighborhoods, and have done that in New Zealand, Paris, Canada, Australia, and every major American city. I just spent eight days in New York City and walked four to eight miles each day—no cabs. I lost weight even eating bagels the size of a tire! Instead of lifting weights, I schlepped my materials. My suitcase contains aerobic shoes, a cap, neck scarf, and sunblock 35. I 'layer' so I can walk in Chicago along the lake in ten degrees and in New Orleans when it is ninety."—Susan RoAne, keynote speaker, author of *How to Work a Room*, *www.susanroane.com*.

Phone on Foot. After a long day, you'll be tempted to lie down on your bed to call loved ones at home or discuss the day with colleagues. But talking on the phone for 30 minutes while lying down burns only 4 calories, while having the same conversation standing up burns 20. Pacing while talking burns even more: 68, even at a slow pace.

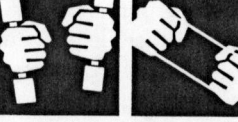
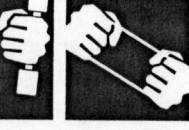

Dyna-Band Hotel Workout. Dyna-Bands are stretchy latex resistance bands that work your muscles as though you're lifting weights. You can pack a set into a pair of shoes in your suitcase, and they weigh practically nothing, so they're perfect traveling companions. Here are some exercises you can do in your hotel room. You'll need one band for most exercises, two bands for some. (See additional Dyna-Band exercises in Chapter 11. See the Resources Appendix for more information about Dyna-Bands.) These exercises are done standing unless otherwise noted.

- **One-Armed Pull-Down.** Stand with your feet hip-width apart, your left hand holding the band about 4 inches above your head. Grasp the band with your right hand just above eye level. Lower both shoulders and keep them lowered, even when your arms are lifted. Pull your right elbow back until your hand is at your shoulder. Squeeze your shoulder blades. Slowly release. Repeat 8 to 12 times before switching sides. This works the large muscles of the back.
- **Open Pull.** Hold your band with your hands about shoulder-width apart, palms up, arms extended straight in front of your chest. Open your arms out to the side until the band touches or almost touches your chest, squeezing your shoulder blades. Slowly return to the starting position. Repeat 8 to 12 times. This works the upper back and shoulders.

- **Bent-Knee Biceps.** Stand with the right leg bent and forward of the left leg. Wrap the band around the back of the right thigh just above the knee. Hold one end of the band in each hand in front of your thigh, palms up. Keeping the elbows into the waist, bend the elbows and pull the hands up to chest level. Slowly return to the starting position. Repeat 8 to 12 times before switching sides. This works the front of the upper arms.
- **Triceps Push-Down.** Hold the band at chest level with your left hand. Grasp the band a few inches away with your right hand, elbow close to your waist. Without moving your left hand, push down with your right hand until your arm is straight. Slowly return to the starting position. Repeat 8 to 12 times before switching sides. This works the back of the upper arms.
- **Inner Thigh Press.** Lie on your back, legs up in the air. Using two bands, wrap one band around each of your inner thighs near the knees, so that the ends emerge at your outer thighs. Hold both ends of one band in each hand. Let your arms extend out to the sides until your hands are touching the floor on either side of your body. This will force your thighs to open. Keeping your hands anchored on the floor, try to press your thighs together, hold for a few seconds, and slowly release to the open position. Repeat 8 to 12 times. This works the inner thighs. Advanced, very flexible: Wrap the bands around your calves rather than your thighs. (Your

thighs will still do the work, but it will be more difficult.)

- **Outer Thigh Press.** Get in the same beginning position as **Inner Thigh Press**, except wrap the bands around your outer thighs so that the ends emerge between your inner thighs. Then cross the bands and switch ends: The right hand holds the ends of the left band, and vice versa. Bring your hands to your chest and anchor them there. Now your thighs are locked closed. Keeping your hands anchored at your chest, try to open your thighs, hold for a few seconds, and slowly release to the closed position. Repeat 8 to 12 times. This works the outer thighs.

Heavy Reading. Sit in a chair holding the phone book. With your feet together, flex your feet (toes up, heels down). Rest the phone book against your shins, balanced on your feet. Slowly straighten your legs, lifting your feet and the book. Slowly return to original position. Repeat 8 to 12 times. Too easy? Use your briefcase, purse, or (packed) duffle bag instead of the phone book.

Jump Rope. The easiest aerobic prop to carry in your suitcase is a jump rope. Use it for frequent, short bouts of cardio—5 minutes in the morning, 5 minutes when you get back to your hotel room at the end of the day, 5 minutes while you're watching the news, and so on. Don't have a jump rope? Pretend you have one, and jump your invisible rope.

Hotel Gym

Hotel gyms range from awesome to icky, and sometimes you can't tell which you'll find until you get there. Even the worst gym, however, will have some basic cardio and strength equipment that works. Use it! If you've got one of the icky gyms, inspect any machines you use and avoid those with warning signs such as frayed cables or rust. Carry your own towel—gym rats (the human kind) are notorious for not noticing when they've left pools of sweat behind. Here are some ways to use the gym:

- **Treadmill:** Set the speed for a comfortable pace for walking or running, starting out slowly to warm up. Be sure you know where the "stop" or "pause" button is before you start so that you can stop quickly if you need to.
- **Stair stepper:** It's like walking upstairs, except you don't get anywhere. Keep your body upright—don't lean on the railing. Try to take big, strong strides rather than baby steps.
- **Stationary bike:** Just sit down and pedal. First, adjust the seat height so that your feet reach the pedals in the "down" position with a very slight bend to the knee.
- **Weight machine (multi-gym):** Illustrated instructions for each weight station should be posted in clear view. If these make sense to you, choose a familiar-looking station and use it first. If the machine works smoothly and comfortably, go ahead and try some other exercises. But if it doesn't feel right, is difficult to adjust to your size or fitness level, or if it has frayed cables, torn seat padding, a jerky feel, or other signs of age and neglect, don't use the machine.
- **Weight bench:** This is used for various dumbbell exercises, but you can also use it for crunches if you don't want to lie on the floor and no one's waiting for the bench.

- **Free weights (dumbbells):** If you know how to use free weights, go ahead, but a hotel gym isn't the place to learn if you haven't. If you're experienced, give yourself a balanced workout of all the major muscle groups—don't just do biceps curls. Hotel gyms often have a limited range of free weights, so you might be frustrated at not finding the amount of weight you need for a particular exercise.

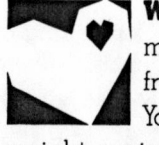 **Walk to a Gym.** Some hotels have an arrangement with a local gym: for a small fee or sometimes free, you can work out where the locals exercise. You'll have access to a full array of cardio and weight equipment and classes.

Swim Off the Day. Most hotels have pools, and what could be more refreshing than a swim at the beginning or end of the day? You'll use more muscles—both upper and lower body—than any other aerobic activity. The rhythm of your strokes and the exertion of your muscles will wash away all the stresses of the day, and the cool temperature of the water will wake you so you can enjoy your day or evening. You'll feel invigorated as well as relaxed. And you'll escape the noise of the city and the chatter of your associates in the peaceful silence of the welcoming water.

Fitness Room Service

Some upscale hotels have fitness equipment or videos that can be delivered to your room for a fee. Some even offer live personal trainers. Ask if these services are available.

 **Dance the Night Away.** Spend an evening dancing in the hotel lounge. Whatever your dancing style or ability, you'll burn calories, de-stress, reenergize, and have a good, sociable time. For more adventure and probably better music, find out where the locals go dancing and go there instead.

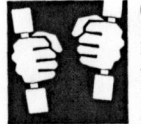 **Chair Your Hamstrings.** Lie on your back on the floor with your left leg extended up, your right leg bent at the knee, and your right heel on the seat of a chair. Push down with your right heel, lifting your lower body off the floor. Let yourself down to the starting position and repeat 8 to 12 times. Repeat with the other leg. Beginners: Keep both heels on the chair. Advanced: Use one heel, and don't let your buttocks touch the floor when you let yourself down. Despite the lack of any equipment except a chair, this is a tough strengthener for your hamstrings (back of thighs).

 **Abs, Abs, Abs.** You don't need anything but the rug to work your abdominal muscles effectively. Try this combination of exercises:

1. **Crunch.** Lie on your back, knees bent. Cross your arms over your chest or place your hands behind your neck, elbows out to the side. Do not pull on your head. Take a deep breath. As you exhale, pull your abdominal muscles in and let that muscle contraction lift your chest, then shoulders, then—if you're strong enough—shoulder blades. Hold at the top for 2 seconds before slowly releasing down for 4 seconds. Keep your head and neck relaxed through the whole sequence. Repeat 8 to 12 times.

2. **Twisting Crunch.** Put the right heel on the left knee. Place your right hand on your right thigh. Start as if you were doing the regular **Crunch**, but when you get halfway up, twist at the waist to the right and continue curling up toward your right knee. Slowly release down. Repeat 8 to 12 times before changing sides.

3. **Reverse Crunch, Advanced.** Lie on your back, legs in the air, arms by your sides, palms down. As you exhale, gently rock your legs toward you and contract your abdominals so that your rear lifts slightly off the ground. Return to starting and repeat 8 to 12 times. Use abdominal

power—don't cheat by pushing hard with your hands or swinging your legs to get the movement started.

One-Legged Bed Squat. Stand at about arm's length away from the side of the bed, facing away from it. Put your right foot on the bed behind you, standing on the left leg. Bending the left leg, lower your body straight down until your left thigh is almost parallel to the floor. If your left knee goes past your toes, you're too close to the bed—hop away until you're the right distance to keep your left knee right above your toes. Repeat 8 to 12 times before changing legs. This works the thighs and buttocks intensely. Be sure to stretch afterwards.

Floor Stretches. Relax at the end of the day with the floor stretches from Chapter 11 for the **chest and shoulders, neck, quadriceps, hamstrings, and buttocks.** Add the **Low-Back Stretch** and the **Cat Stretch** (p. 214).

Low-Back Stretch. Lie on your back, knees bent. Bring the right knee up toward your chest until you can hook your arm underneath it. Pull the leg in closer until you feel your lower back stretch. If it's comfortable, extend the left leg straight on the floor. Repeat with the other side. For a more intense stretch, pull both legs in toward your chest at the same time, clasping your hands behind your knees. (If you can't reach, use a towel behind your knees and hold on to both ends.) This is an excellent stretch whenever your lower back feels tight and especially following abdominal exercises.

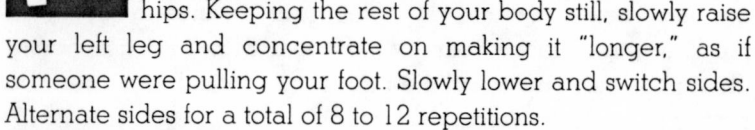

Low-Back Strengthener. Lie on your stomach on the floor, your chin resting on your hands, both legs straight on the floor and open a little wider than your hips. Keeping the rest of your body still, slowly raise your left leg and concentrate on making it "longer," as if someone were pulling your foot. Slowly lower and switch sides. Alternate sides for a total of 8 to 12 repetitions.

Low-Back Strengthener, Variation. Lie on your stomach on the floor, your arms extended in front of you. Do **Low-Back Strengthener** above, but extend and lift the right arm as you lift the left leg, and vice versa.

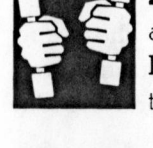

Cat Stretch. Release back and neck tension at the end of the day with this stretch on the hotel room rug. Get on hands and knees, back neutral. Imagine that a string attached to the back of your waist is pulling you up as you round your back slowly, letting your head drop forward. Hold for a few seconds, then let the back sink slowly into an arch, chin up. Slowly alternate between the two positions 4 to 6 times. Finish by letting your hips fall toward your feet, your back rounded over your knees, your face to one side on the rug (you might want a clean towel under it), your arms resting comfortably at your sides, palms up. Relax there.

12

Chapter 17

9   **Getting It**   3
            Together:
      Playing It Safe

6

T
HE SAFEST WAY TO EXERCISE is exactly what we're recommending here: short bouts of physical activity designed to fit your individual pace and comfort. Even so, we're all different, and you need to make sure your fitness activities are right for your age, weight, fitness level, and overall health. If you have any medical conditions that might be affected by your exercise program, please consult your physician and follow his or her recommendations.

Beyond choosing the right exercises, you'll benefit from learning how to do them correctly, so we've gathered guidelines for safe stretching, stepping, and weightlifting. You'll also learn some **217** safety tips ranging from cautions about child carriers to avoiding heat stroke to protecting yourself from bad guys when you're walking outdoors. We want you to be safe as well as fit and healthy.

Your Target Heart Rate

You've heard that you're supposed to condition your heart and lungs with aerobic exercise, but how can you tell if you're exercising at the right intensity? For aerobic exercise, you're aiming for an intensity that brings your heart rate into a certain range called the "target heart-rate zone." In other words, you want to raise your heart rate to a certain number of beats per minute to qualify as aerobic. But you don't want to go over that range, especially if you're a beginning exerciser. Here's how to figure out your personal target heart rate (THR) zone, according to the American Heart Association:

1. Subtract your age from 220. This is your maximum heart rate. 220 minus your age = _____.
2. Multiply your answer to #1 by 50% = _____.
3. Multiply your answer to #1 by 75% = _____.

Your THR zone is the range between your answer to #2 and your answer to #3. For example, if you're 50 years old, your maximum heart rate is 170 and your target heart-rate zone is 85 to 127.

To find out how intensely you're exercising, get to the exercise peak where you feel you're breathing harder, sweating, feeling warm. Stop moving and quickly take your pulse, counting the beats for 10 seconds and multiplying by 6. Are you in the zone?

If you're a beginning exerciser, overweight, or have a medical condition that limits your exercise intensity, stay closer to the 50 percent mark. You should be able to talk in complete sentences without gasping. If you're an athlete or a seasoned, well-conditioned exerciser, you can work out harder—substitute 65 percent for #2 and 85 percent for #3 in the formula.

Drink Your Water

Not only is water necessary for life, it is essential for looking and feeling your best. Drinking enough water will help you avoid lethargy, dry skin, headaches, constipation, and lack of mental clarity—all possible signs of dehydration.

Don't wait until you feel thirsty before you reach for your water bottle because by then you may already be somewhat dehydrated. How much water is enough? Here are some easy guidelines:

- Eight 8-ounce glasses of water daily is the standard recommendation. (See "Your Personal Water Calculation," following.)

- Drink extra water when you exercise: 2 cups before exercising and more every 15 to 20 minutes while you work out.
- Drink extra water in hot, humid, or cold weather or high altitudes; when flying; and if you have a cold, flu, or fever.
- Water is your best fluid source. Milk and juices are okay, too. Caffeinated beverages and alcohol, however, increase fluid loss (they act as diuretics, medicines which make you urinate more than you are taking in). Have an extra glass of water for each cup of these liquids that you drink.
- Start each day with a glass of water when you get up, one midmorning, one or two during the afternoon, one with each meal, and one at night. Keep a water bottle in the car and on your desk at work.

Your Personal Water Calculation

Although eight 8-ounce glasses of water daily is the standard recommendation, you, personally, might need more, especially if you exercise. IDEA Health and Fitness Association, the international organization of health and fitness professionals, offers this way to calculate your personal fluid needs:

1. Divide your weight in half. This number in ounces is your recommended daily water intake.
2. Divide that number by 8 to figure out the number of 8-ounce glasses.

Here's an example to walk you through the math: You weigh 180 pounds.

1. One-half of 180 is 90, the ounces of water you should consume.
2. Ninety divided by 8 equals 11¼ glasses of water.

Now you do it:

1. My weight is _____.
2. One-half of my weight is _____, the ounces of water I should consume.
3. The ounces divided by 8 equals _____ 8-ounce glasses of water.

How to Work Out with a Video

For safety, comfort, effectiveness, and enjoyment, follow these guidelines when exercising with an aerobic workout video.

- Watch the whole workout before doing it. Notice the body alignment of the leader and listen to the directions. Learn which cues match which moves.
- Don't be impatient to learn the whole workout the first time you do it. Pause, rewind, and figure out the moves as you go. Just do the footwork while you're learning. Add the arms later.
- Follow the modifications for your fitness level.
- Stay within your target heart-rate range. Most videos take

you through a heart-rate check. If not, you do the "talk test": You should be able to talk in complete sentences without gasping, but you might be exercising too hard to sing.

- Just do part of the workout if you don't have the stamina to do the whole thing. When you're ready to quit, fast-forward to the cool-down/stretch segment. Always start from the beginning so you get an appropriate warm-up.
- Don't do anything that hurts, especially if it hurts your back or joints. Make sure you're doing the move properly—sometimes a simple adjustment in back alignment or knee position will make all the difference. If not, don't do the move at all.

Safe Stepping

Step aerobics is great exercise, combining an intense cardiovascular, low-impact workout with lower-body strengthening. If you plan to exercise to a step video, invest in a commercial step platform. You can build a wooden step cheaply, but this isn't as resilient or safe, and you can cut your leg on the corners if you fall. In contrast, the commercial step has a slip-proof tread and rounded corners.

Commercial platforms let you adjust the height of the step. The higher the step, the harder the workout. Start out at the lowest level (just the platform with no risers), then add height as you feel secure and need more intensity. Don't rush to add height—you can get a superb workout with the platform at its lowest level.

If you're stepping at home to a videotape, set up a full-length mirror right beside the television, if you can, so you can watch the video and your feet (in the mirror) at the same time. While you're learning, stick to the most basic step workout (often free with your step purchase) until you know where your feet are on the step without looking and you understand the movements and cueing. Until you feel very secure, avoid movements that turn you around so you're not facing the video.

Safe Stretching

The point of stretching is to release muscle tension and increase flexibility and range of movement within your personal limits. Stretching the muscles after working them is especially helpful. Avoid "ballistic" stretches that use fast, forceful, jerky, or bouncy motions. Muscles react to sudden, exaggerated stretching by tightening instead of relaxing. Use slow, static stretches, where you relax into the stretch, breathing deeply, sinking a little farther each time you exhale. Other safe stretching tips:

- Never force a stretch beyond your comfortable limit.
- If a stretch causes discomfort, omit it.
- Never bounce or force a stretch.

- If you can't reach the limb you're stretching, don't force it— use a towel around your leg or foot (depending on what you're trying to reach) to extend your reach.
- Never stretch beyond your personal, comfortable limits.

=============== **To Stretch or Not to Stretch** ===============

Some medical conditions may be worsened by stretching. Do not stretch without your physician's clearance if you have any of these conditions:

- Recent bone fracture.
- Acute inflammation or infection around a joint.
- Sharp, acute pain with joint movement or muscle lengthening.
- Recent sprain (ligament injury) or strain (muscle or tendon injury).
- Muscle injury.

Weightlifting Basics

Whether you're weight training with free weights (dumbbells), a weight machine, or resistance bands, form and technique are crucial for getting a safe and effective workout. Follow these guidelines:

- Warm up the muscles you're going to use, going through a sampler of the muscle movements you're planning, but without weights. Or do 5 to 10 minutes of an all-purpose exercise that warms up all your muscles, such as brisk walking.

- Perform all movements slowly, using a 6-second repetition or even slower. Don't rush to the end of a move. Rather, feel the move every inch of the way. Return to your starting position even more slowly than you left it—don't just let go.
- Work through the full range of motion recommended for each exercise. Don't shorten the move or just do the part that's easy.
- Breathe! Exhale on the lifting or pulling phase; inhale when lowering or releasing. Don't hold your breath.
- Keep the resistance difficult to make the fastest progress. Choose a weight or intensity at which you can perform only 8 to 12 repetitions in slow, controlled, proper form. Your muscle should be quite tired before 12. Once you can do 12 repetitions in good form, increase the weight or resistance slightly so that you can do only 8.
- Stretch each muscle group you've worked after you're done.
- Strength-train 2 or 3 times a week, and don't work the same muscles on consecutive days.
- No pain. Don't overdo it. Mild soreness the next day—a slight ache or stiffness—just means your muscles are adapting, and it will pass. But if you're feeling pain that interferes with your day, you overdid it.
- Tune in to how your body feels at all times. If a move hurts, don't do it. Pain in the joints, such as knee pain, means something is wrong. Check your technique carefully. If your

technique is right and you still experience joint pain, stop and do a different exercise that doesn't cause pain. Be careful of previous injuries. Test an injured area with no weight or light weight. If there's any pain, stop.

- Treat old injury sites with special care. Those areas may not be as strong as before, even though you think they're completely healed. Get medical advice about rehabilitation exercises if you find you have these weak or sensitive spots.

Hot Exercise

Be cautious exercising in the heat. The American College of Sports Medicine (ACSM) advises that you exercise in the cooler hours of morning and evening, if possible. If you must exercise outdoors in the heat, the ACSM recommends these precautions to prevent heat exhaustion and heat stroke:

- Avoid dehydration by drinking plenty of liquids, enough fluid to replace sweat loss: 5 to 10 ounces every 15 minutes. Weigh yourself before and after your workout—if you weigh the same, you've replenished your fluid adequately. (No, the weight loss isn't fat loss—not this fast, sorry!)
- Wear lightweight, loose-fitting clothing to allow sweat to evaporate and cool the body.
- Acclimatize yourself to the heat by starting out with very short

sessions at very light intensity and gradually increasing the duration and intensity over 10 to 14 days.

- If you have an ongoing illness, respiratory infection, diarrhea, vomiting, or fever, don't exercise in the heat.

═ Heat Exhaustion, Heat Stroke—What's the Difference? ═

Heat exhaustion is caused by becoming overheated and dehydrated. Symptoms may include dizziness, weakness, nausea, vomiting, muscle aches, and headache. It usually can be treated with cooling, rest, and fluids, but sometimes—especially when nausea and vomiting are present—medical care and intravenous fluid replacement are needed. Heat exhaustion is a relatively benign condition, if treated properly.

Heat stroke is a serious medical emergency that can be fatal. Heat stroke occurs when the body's internal mechanisms fail to cool the body. Sweating stops (not always immediately) and the body temperature rises beyond normal limits. If body temperature exceeds 108°F, brain damage may occur. Since it is not always easy to tell the difference, seek medical help immediately unless the affected person is drinking liquids and cooling down quickly. Call for an ambulance if the person cannot retain fluids or seems to be getting worse when brought to a cool environment, especially if he or she is not sweating or is acting confused. First-aid measures include sponging or spraying the skin with cool water and hastening evaporation with fans while waiting for the ambulance. Some medical professionals advocate also putting ice packs in the armpits and groin, but the evaporation is more important. Aspirin and Tylenol do not help.

But I Don't Feel Well

Should you exercise if you're not feeling well? It depends. If you're ill or coming down with an illness, it's better to rest. If you feel as if some exertion would clear your stuffy head or relieve your stiff muscles, the rule of thumb (or, in this case, "rule of neck") is that if your illness is above the neck, mild exercise won't do any harm and might make you feel better. If it's below the neck, though, better to just rest. Absolutely do not exercise if you have muscle aches, a fever of 100°F or higher, chills, diarrhea, a hacking cough, or vomiting.

If you have "above the neck" symptoms and you decide to exercise, don't push it. Do light exercise—maybe half as much as you're used to and slower than your usual pace. If getting your body moving starts making you feel better within the first few minutes, continue. If it doesn't, stop. Take a relaxing bath. Go to bed with a good book. Drink plenty of fluids. Your body requires energy to fight off illness, so this is definitely *not* the time to work on increasing your aerobic endurance. Becoming over-tired from excessive exercise may slow your recovery time. If you feel you have little energy, do some gentle stretching rather than aerobic or muscle-strengthening workouts. Take it easy.

When you feel better and decide to get back into exercise, keep your exercise light and work back to your normal routine very gradually.

Child on Board

Is it safe to take young children with you on grown-up walks, jogs, and bike rides with jogging strollers, bike seats or trailers, or backpacks? Experts differ about safety, but recommend these cautions if you plan to do it:

- Stick to familiar routes with a smooth running surface and little or no traffic.
- Avoid terrains with potholes, cracks, or rocks.
- Make sure your child's clothing is right for the temperature and wind conditions. Use sun block.
- Keep your mind alert and focused on your child's safety.
- Buy a sturdy, stable jogging stroller that does not tip on a turn. Make sure it fits your child and has a locking brake.
- Do not take a child in a bike seat unless you're an expert cyclist because the child's weight and the seat add instability to the bike (which is unstable on its own). The child should be old enough to hold up his or her head.
- A bike trailer is safer than a bike seat, but the ride is rougher on the child and maneuverability is more difficult.
- If you bicycle with a child, both of you should wear helmets.
- Never wear a baby backpack when doing activities with risk of a fall, such as skiing, or near moving equipment, such as lawn mowing.

Road Safety

If you walk or jog after dark, be aware of how difficult it is for drivers to see you. Even though you can see the car, the driver might not be able to see you until it's too late to stop or swerve. Protect yourself by wearing reflective markings—available at sporting goods stores—to make yourself more visible. Attach them at all your major joints: wrists, elbows, knees, shoulders, hips, and ankles. This way the driver not only sees you, but identifies you as a moving person.

Self-Protection Strategies

It's horrible to think that you have to anticipate protecting yourself against people who want to do you harm while you're exercising outdoors, but it's reality. Better to think out your strategies ahead of time and never need them than to avoid the subject and be unprepared when you're in danger.

John Martin, president and cofounder of Combat Arts Institute in Palatine, Illinois (*www.combatarts.org*), cautions you to stay aware of your surroundings—not just traffic and terrain, but also the people. Be wary of people behaving strangely or showing facial expressions or mannerisms that aren't right—clenched fist, sweating while standing still, or furtive glances, for example. Stay clear of any person who makes you feel uncomfortable or fearful, even if there's no logical reason for your feeling.

Think before you stop to answer questions or offer help. Usually someone who asks the time or directions is another well-meaning person enjoying the trail or park—but someone who means you harm will often use this ruse to make you stop and get you off guard. Assess before answering, and answer without stopping.

If your gut feeling is that something isn't right, trust it. If anything makes you queasy or uneasy, don't stop. Your brain is capable of receiving signals that something is wrong before you can analyze the reason. "Acknowledge that your gut instinct is an indicator light—sometimes it will be wrong, but the higher risk is ignoring it when it's real," says Martin.

Martin offers these additional tips for staying safe:

- Know where you're going and what to expect. Know your environment before you go.
- Leave a way for someone else to track you. Let someone know your plan and your schedule.
- If you live alone, record a memo on your answering machine or leave a note at your front door telling when you're going, where, and when you expect to be back.
- If you carry your cell phone so you can call for help, practice using it without looking at it.
- Do not rely on defensive strategies—like pepper spray or other self-defense devices—that you haven't been trained to

use and practiced many times. Make sure anything you're carrying for defense is accessible—in your hand or ready to grasp in an instant, not in your back pocket or fanny pack.

- Know your escape route. What would you do if you were being chased? Where would you go to find safety? Run through this mentally.
- Don't wear a headset that either blocks outside sound or distracts you so that you're not paying attention. Stay receptive to warning sounds.
- Look at people's faces, but not directly into their eyes, which can be perceived as challenging. Look at their chins, noses, hands, feet, and clothing. Look for about a second—don't stare. If you don't look at all, it's a sign of fearfulness. If you look too long, it's a challenge.
- Scream "No! No! No!" if attacked or threatened. Don't yell "Help!" because many people are not willing to risk their own well-being to put themselves in an unknown danger. Yelling "No!" conveys that something bad is happening but doesn't sound as threatening as "Help!" and people are more likely to come out to investigate.
- Take some sort of training in how to break away from attacks.
- Walk with a few friends. It will make the walk more enjoyable and safer.

12

Chapter 18

9   **Quick
Gym Visits**   3

6

I

T DOESN'T DO ANY GOOD TO GO TO THE GYM if you just have a
few minutes, right? Wrong! Even a 5- to 10-minute gym
workout invigorates you and gives you the opportunity to
use some equipment you don't have at home, such as an aerobic step, stability ball, Gravitron, rower, or elliptical trainer.
And you can use the free weights or weight machines to
strengthen two muscle groups in less than 5 minutes, including
the stretch afterwards.   **233**

Cardio Circuit. Do you get bored on cardio machines? Choose a variety—exercise bike, stair machine, elliptical trainer, rower, treadmill—and do just 5 minutes on one machine, then quickly switch to another. Depending on how much time you spend total, you'll not only burn calories and condition your heart and lungs, but also work a variety of muscles because each machine targets your muscles differently.

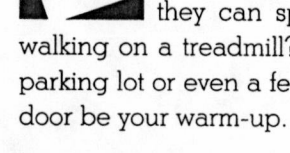

Parking Solution. Haven't you seen people circle around in their cars, trying to get a parking space as close as possible to the health club's front door so that they can spend 30 minutes climbing fake stairs or walking on a treadmill? Duh! Park at the farthest recesses of the parking lot or even a few blocks away, and let the trek to the front door be your warm-up.

Step Fit. An aerobic step is a great prop to give you an intense, sweaty, aerobic workout. Every riser level you add increases intensity and calorie burning. If you're a beginner, take a class rather than trying to figure it out on your own. Start with no risers (4-inch step) or one set of risers (6-inch step). If you've been stepping for a while and you don't get out of breath at your present level, challenge yourself with another set of risers. A 120-pound person doing basic stepping (nothing fancy, no armwork) for 10 minutes at 120 beats per minute will burn 45 calories on a 4-inch step, 55 calories at 6 inches, 64 at 8 inches, and 72 at 10 inches. If you want to add intensity, go higher rather than faster. Stepping at too fast of a pace doesn't allow your heels to come all the way down, putting you at increased risk of injury. And please warm up first! See Chapter 17 for more about step aerobics.

Row, Row, Row Off Calories. The rowing machine is one of the most effective cardio machines because it uses both upper- and lower-body muscles. It particularly targets the large muscles of the back, which is unusual for a cardio machine. A 150-pound person burns between 80 and 136 calories in just 10 minutes of rowing. Although correct rowing technique sounds complicated, it will become natural very quickly. Here's how to use the rower correctly:

1. Start with your knees bent, shins as close to perpendicular to the floor as your flexibility permits, your back neutral and leaning slightly forward from the hips.
2. Push with your legs, then swing back with your upper body and pull the handle into your abdomen as you straighten your legs, leaning back slightly.
3. Let your arms lengthen, lean forward from the hips, bend your legs, and slide forward (in that order) until you're in starting position to take the next stroke.

People sure are working up a sweat on those big, shiny cardio machines, but when you timidly approach for the first time, you're likely to skitter away intimidated. There are all these settings to program—how's a gal or guy to know?

A good club should offer an initial training session when you join. Ask. If you've been a member for a while and you're too embarrassed to admit that you've never tried the machine that intrigues you now, here are some tips from the IDEA Health & Fitness Association (*www.ideafit.com*), the international organization of health and fitness professionals, for using a cardio machine for the first time:

- **Know how to stop.** Before you begin, learn how to stop the equipment in case you need to get off quickly. Look for a "stop" or "pause" button on the console or a safety switch. Some machines slow to a halt when you stop moving.
- **Start simply.** Your first time, just do the manual or steady-state program without trying the more complex settings. A manual program lets you adjust the intensity, incline, and speed as you go. A steady-state program gives you a warm-up, a cardio workout, and a cool-down.
- **Understand the options.** Many machines have preset or individually set programs that control your speed, intensity, duration, and/or incline. Read the instructions on the console to see how to set these. If these seem too complicated, go back to the manual program.
- **Try an interval program.** Most machines these days have preset interval programs that alternate periods of harder and lighter intensity. These may be called "fat burning" or "weight loss" programs.

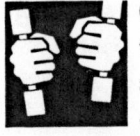 **Gravitron Quickie.** The Gravitron is a strength-training machine designed to put you through a series of exercises for all the major upper-body muscles. You stand on the platform, and then punch in your weight and intensity level. The platform rises as you do a variety of pull-ups and triceps dips, with the machine "assisting" you a little or a lot, depending on which level you choose. You can get a quick workout by following the directions for sets and repetitions printed on the machine, or even quicker by doing just one set of each exercise. To make this effective, be sure to choose an intensity difficult enough to fatigue your muscles in one set, but not so difficult that you can't perform the exercises.

Something New. Try a machine you've never tried before. The elliptical trainer (also called cross-trainer), for example, is a cool cardio machine that lets you walk in an inclined egg-shape motion, targeting the hamstrings and buttocks more than most cardio machines. The description sounds weird, but it's a very comfortable and unusual workout, sort of a cross between a ski machine and a stair machine.

If you feel motivated when you're around fitness-oriented people and activities and especially if you might enjoy classes or having your choice of a variety of expensive, well-maintained exercise equipment, joining a fitness club (also known as health club or gym) might appeal to you. But realize that the club you choose can make or break your best intentions.

Clubs vary widely in the equipment, classes, activities, and amenities they offer, as well as what they charge. A club membership will work for you only if you feel at ease there and want to show up. Here are some guidelines:

- Make a list of what you want from a fitness club, including equipment, ambience, classes, location, and cost.
- Phone different clubs to find out about costs.
- Be wary of clubs that offer a price for "today only" or lifetime memberships for a suspiciously low price. They may mean their "lifetime" rather than yours and plan to close soon, or they may make it impossible to cancel.
- Be wary of clubs that consistently and substantially undercut their competitors. They may hire cheap and untrained help, buy inferior equipment, and ignore members.
- Emphasize convenience. It won't do you any good to join an inexpensive club on the other side of town if you won't go there. Be sure the location and hours fit your needs. Studies have shown that if you live or work within a 15-minute drive, you're more likely to get there consistently.
- Visit the clubs that pass your initial screening. Spend an hour or so at each one, not just taking the "guided tour," but also checking

out the classes, equipment, cleanliness of the locker room, and so on. Is the club clean, especially the showers and locker room? Is the equipment well maintained? Are members getting instruction and attention as they use the equipment? Time your visit so you're there during the hours you would attend if you joined to see how crowded the club is at that time and what classes are offered. Some clubs will issue day passes to potential members, permitting you to work out at the club and try the classes.

- Ask members about what they like and dislike about the club. Don't interrupt someone who's working out—instead, converse in the locker room, which is often a friendly and social place.
- Ask yourself if you feel comfortable in the club's atmosphere. Can you picture yourself working out there?
- Don't sign anything until you've had time to go home and think about it and you're satisfied that this club is for you. Get all the information about costs, payment plans, setup or initiation fee, cancellation, and discounts (for couples, families, seniors, whatever fits). Resist any pressure—do not sign up until and unless you're sure.

Walking Lunge. You can get a fast lower-body strengthening workout by holding a barbell or Body Bar on your shoulders and lunge-walking across the room. Take a huge step forward with your right leg, bending both knees as you land, your right thigh ending up parallel to the floor and your right knee positioned over your arch, not forward of your toes. Push up to standing and do the same with the left leg. By the time you travel across the room, your thighs and buttocks should be burning.

Ball Crunches. Sit on a stability ball (those colorful, thigh-high balls at many health clubs). Choose a size that permits you to sit on it with your knees making a right angle. Lower your back onto the ball as you inch your feet away, rolling the ball along your back until your lower back is supported. Do slow abdominal crunches from this position. The ball lets you release lower than you could on the floor, increasing the range of motion and, therefore, difficulty and effectiveness. Keep your feet wide apart to help you stabilize until you're experienced with the ball.

Advanced Ball Crunches. Do Ball Crunches above, but keep your feet very close together to give yourself more of a stability challenge. This makes the balancing more difficult, and you have to activate the core muscles of the abdominals and back to keep from rolling off the ball.

Ball Push-Ups. Kneel on the floor and wrap your arms and upper body over a stability ball. Now straighten your legs, pushing yourself over the rolling ball until you're draped over the ball, hands touching the floor. Now "walk" your hands away from the ball until your legs are on the ball, your back is straight, and your upper body is suspended. This is your starting position. Tighten your abdominals to stabilize, and do push-ups from this position. You'll not only get a good upper-body workout, but your abdominals and back will work hard to keep you in position.

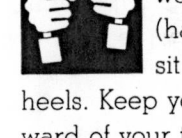 **Dumbbell Squats.** Stand up straight, your heavier weights at your sides (easier) or on your shoulders (harder). Slowly lower your body as if you're about to sit in a chair, keeping your body weight over your heels. Keep your back neutral. Do not let your knees travel forward of your toes. Squeeze your buttocks as you straighten up. Sit back to keep your knees over your arch, not past your toes. Repeat 8 to 12 times. This strengthens your thighs and buttocks.

Bent-Over Dumbbell Row. Stand on your left leg, with your right knee on a weight bench. Bend forward from your hips so that your back is parallel to the bench. Rest your right hand on the bench and hold one of your heavier weights in your left hand, arm extended down and perpendicular to the bench. Roll your shoulder back. Contract your back muscles while bringing the weight toward your rib cage, letting your elbow flare out and keeping the weight close to your body. Squeeze your shoulder blades. Slowly lower. Keep your abdominals tight, back neutral. Repeat 8 to 12 times. Change sides. This works the large muscles of the back.

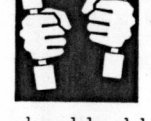 **Dumbbell Shrug.** Stand holding your heavier weights, feet hip-width apart, arms at your sides holding your heavier weights, shoulders relaxed. Lift your shoulders to your ears in a shrugging movement. Concentrate on squeezing your shoulder blades. Hold for a few seconds, then slowly release to the starting position. Repeat 8 to 12 times. This upper-back strengthener is also an effective stress-reliever for upper-back tension.

Dumbbell Upright Row. Stand up straight, holding your lighter weights in your hands in front of your thighs. Lift your arms up along your body, elbows out to the side, stopping at your chest. Squeeze your shoulder blades, pulling your elbows back. Lift and lower 8 to 12 times. This strengthens your upper back.

Dumbbell Chest Press. Lie on your back on a weight bench, feet flat on the floor or bench, depending on your height. (Your back should not arch.) Hold your heavier weights in your hands at your shoulders. Slowly push your arms straight up above your chest. Hold for a moment, then slowly release. Be careful not to arch your back or lock your elbows. Lift and lower 8 to 12 times. This exercise strengthens the chest.

How Heavy?

We're sure you've noticed that when we describe a dumbbell exercise, we don't tell you how heavy the weight should be—we just say "lighter" or "heavier." That's because the actual poundage depends on how strong you are. It would be a disservice to tell you to lift 5 pounds when you're capable of lifting 15 pounds in perfect form. Likewise, you could get hurt by trying to lift 15 pounds if your comfortable limit is 10 pounds. And since some of your muscles are much stronger than others, you'll need different weights for different muscle groups.

Here's how to figure out the right amount of weight to use:

1. Start with the **Dumbbell Biceps Curl** (following). Try out different weights until you find the one that lets you do 8 to 12 repetitions in good form (keeping the back neutral and the body still, no arching or swinging!), but no more than 12. The weight should feel very heavy on your last couple of repetitions. That's your lighter weight.

2. Now take a weight that's quite a bit heavier, anywhere from a few pounds heavier to twice as heavy. Now do your **Bent-Over Dumbbell Row** (p. 241) with this weight. Adjust a little easier or harder until you find the weight that you can lift 8 to12 times in good form. Again, your last repetitions should be very difficult. That's your heavier weight.

3. If you're a woman, your triceps (back of upper arms) and deltoids (shoulders) are proportionately weaker and smaller, and you'll probably need to use weights that are a few pounds lighter than your "lighter" weights.

(Please read Chapter 17 before your first trip to the gym, especially if you're new to lifting weights.)

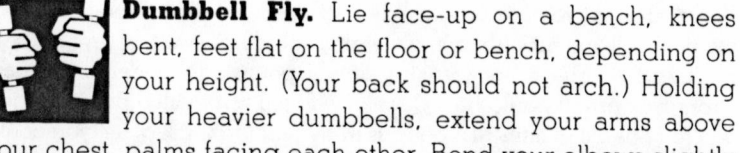

Dumbbell Fly. Lie face-up on a bench, knees bent, feet flat on the floor or bench, depending on your height. (Your back should not arch.) Holding your heavier dumbbells, extend your arms above your chest, palms facing each other. Bend your elbows slightly outward and slowly open your arms, drawing the two sides of a half-circle in the air. Stop when your elbows are at bench level or barely lower than the bench. Contracting your chest muscles, push the dumbbells up and together, returning to the starting position. Lift and lower 8 to 12 times. This exercise strengthens the chest and shoulders.

Dumbbell Biceps Curl. Stand holding your lighter weights at your sides, palms up, elbows at your waist. Slowly lift your weights to your shoulders, keeping your elbows at your waist. Lift and lower 8 to 12 times. This works the front of the upper arm.

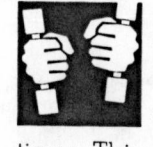

Dumbbell Overhead Triceps. Stand holding one lighter weight in your right hand, your right arm raised at the side of your head, elbow bent so your hand is behind your head. For safety (to keep yourself from clunking yourself in the head), put the left forearm across your forehead, palm out, and hold on to the right upper arm, keeping it still. Slowly straighten your right arm, keeping it beside your head. Avoid arching your back. Bend and straighten 8 to 12 times, then change arms. This works the back of the upper arm.

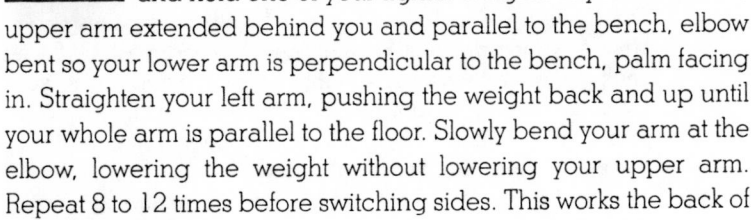 **Dumbbell Triceps Kickback.** Stand on your left leg with your right knee on the bench. Your back is parallel to the bench. Rest your right hand on the bench and hold one of your lighter weights in your left hand, upper arm extended behind you and parallel to the bench, elbow bent so your lower arm is perpendicular to the bench, palm facing in. Straighten your left arm, pushing the weight back and up until your whole arm is parallel to the floor. Slowly bend your arm at the elbow, lowering the weight without lowering your upper arm. Repeat 8 to 12 times before switching sides. This works the back of the upper arm.

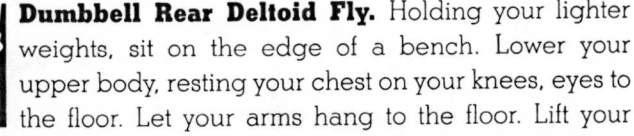 **Dumbbell Rear Deltoid Fly.** Holding your lighter weights, sit on the edge of a bench. Lower your upper body, resting your chest on your knees, eyes to the floor. Let your arms hang to the floor. Lift your arms straight out to the side. Keep your elbows unlocked, but barely bent. Concentrate on keeping your chest lowered to your knees and lifting with the back of the shoulders. The backs of the shoulders are small, weak muscles, and you'll probably need to lighten your weights.

Take 10

This mini-circuit routine alternates aerobics and strength training to provide a full-body workout in just 10 minutes. You need two sets of weights, one set heavier than the other. (The actual weight will vary according to your fitness level and experience.) Do the following moves in order without resting. Put down your weights when you switch to aerobic moves, keeping them within easy reach but not underfoot.

1. March in place and swing your arms for 1 minute to warm up. Then pick up your lighter weights. Hold them palms down, arms at your side, feet parallel and hip-width apart. Squat back, keeping your body weight over your heels, lifting your arms in front to shoulder height (front shoulder raise). Lower your arms as your body rises, and squeeze your buttocks. Repeat 10 times. Put the weights down.

2. March with your knees high or jog for 1 minute. Stop jogging and pick up your heavier weights. Hold them with your arms lowered, the weights touching in front of your thighs, legs wide apart and opened to the diagonal. Lower your buttocks and bend your knees in a wide-legged squat, lifting the weights close to the front of your body, elbows bent, to chest height (upright row). Sit back, not straight down. Lower the weights as your body rises. Repeat 10 times. Put the weights down.

3. March or jog 3 steps, then lift your knee. Repeat "1-2-3-knee up" in place, then forward and back. Repeat for 90 seconds. Then stand with your arms at your side holding the lighter weights, your palms out, feet parallel and hip-width apart. Rise onto the balls of your feet while bringing the weights toward your shoulders (biceps curls), keeping your elbows at

The Anytime, Anywhere Exercise Book

your waist. Rise straight up without rocking forward or back. Lower the weights and your body. Repeat 10 times. Put the weights down.

4. Jump rope, jog, or dance for 90 seconds. Then stand with your feet parallel and hip-width apart, holding the lighter weights. Bend your knees slightly and lean your body forward from the hips, keeping your back neutral. Raise your elbows behind you. Straighten your arms behind you, pushing the weights back (Triceps Kickbacks), then bend. Repeat 10 times.

Dumbbell Deltoid Lateral Raise. Stand or sit with your lighter weights in front of your hips, arms slightly bent. Keeping your shoulders down, lift your arms out to the sides and up to shoulder height, keeping your elbows slightly bent. Lift and lower 8 to 12 times. This works the shoulders.

It's-Too-Nice-a-Day-to-Go-to-the-Gym. Start 1 to 2 miles away from any gym (it doesn't have to be yours). Speedwalk to the gym, slap the wall, turn around, and speedwalk back to your starting place. This works just dandy when the gym is closed or when you're not a gym member. (This even works with a library, courthouse, or doctor's office.) If the gym happens to be open and you happen to be a member, go in, refill your water bottle, and use the restroom before returning to your starting place.

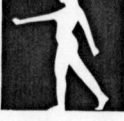 **After-Workout Stretch.** Don't leave the gym without stretching the muscles you just worked. You'll need to find something sturdy you can pull and push on and get your hands around, such as a pole-like, upright section of a sturdy weight machine or a railing. (For simplicity, we'll call it "the railing" in the instructions below.) Choose the specific stretches that fit the workout you did, or do the whole stretch series to feel really great. Hold 10 to 60 seconds in each position.

- **Back and Arms.** Stand an arm's length away from the railing. Lean forward at the waist and hold on to the railing, slightly bending your knees, pushing your weight behind you, and rounding your back.
- **Chest and Shoulders.** Turn around so your back is toward the railing and you're holding on to it behind you. Roll your shoulders back and lean your body forward away from the railing, chest thrust forward.
- **Calves.** Face the railing and hold it with both hands, standing close to it. Bend the left leg slightly as you step the right leg back as far as it can go with the heel pressed down. You'll feel a stretch in the right calf. Then bring the right leg forward a few inches and slightly bend the right knee, keeping the heel down. You'll feel the stretch go lower in the calf. Repeat both positions with the left leg.

- **Quads.** Face the railing and hold it with the left hand. Reach back with the right hand and bend the right knee with the foot behind you until you can hold on to your right ankle (or sock or pant leg, if you can't reach the ankle). Try to keep the thighs together and straighten the back. You'll feel the stretch in the front of the right thigh. Repeat with the left leg.
- **Hip Flexors.** Step back with the right leg. Keeping the left knee bent and directly over the ankle, slide the right leg back until you sink into a lunge, right toes on the ground, right heel lifted. Bend the right knee just to your point of comfort. Don't let the left knee go forward of the foot to avoid stress to the knee. Change legs.
- **Hamstrings.** Stand up straight holding the railing. Straighten and extend the right leg in front of you, flexing the foot (heel down, toes up). Your left leg is slightly bent. Lean forward until you feel the stretch in the right hamstring (back of the thigh). Repeat with the left leg.
- **Buttocks.** Hold the railing with both hands, knees slightly bent. Place the right foot on the left thigh. Bend the left leg a little more, leaning your derrière back as if you were about to sit down. You'll feel the stretch in the right buttock. Change sides.

Quick Gym Visits

249

12

Chapter 19

9 **Exercises to Do 3
While Doing
Something Else**

6

G RANTED, MOST OF THESE ACTIVITIES take more than 5 minutes; some take 30 minutes, 1 hour, or even all day. But
they belong in this book because they really don't take
any extra time; you do them while you're accomplishing something else. Think of it—you can get your exercise done at the
same time as your housework, or you can work out while you
study, "write" letters, garden, or watch television. Here's how. **251**

Letter Aerobics. Are you bored with your indoor cardio equipment? Do you feel guilty because you owe letters to countless friends and family members? Audio-tape letters instead of writing them. Get on the exercise bike, treadmill, or stair machine with your tape recorder in hand or set on the magazine rack, get moving, and tape your news and views as you work out. More fun than laborious writing, this lets you accomplish two things at once, and your tape will be a treat for your friends and relatives to receive. Encourage your correspondents to tape back instead of write, and only listen to their "letters" when you're exercising.

Garage Clean-Up. You say your garage is so crowded that you have to leave your car outside? Spend a Saturday cleaning out and organizing all those piles and boxes. Get rid of everything you can do without (recycling the recyclables, of course), including those toys you meant to repair (your kids are now in graduate school), rusted kitchenware, letters from the sweetie who broke your heart a decade ago, mildewed shoes, and anything else you'd be embarrassed to have anyone know you kept. Once you clear out everything you don't need, sort and organize what's left. You'll be surprised how many muscles you use getting rid of stuff and putting what's left back on nicely

organized shelves.

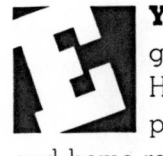 **Yard Work and Home Repair.** No need to go to the gym when you've got a yard or house to maintain. Here's a sampling of how many calories a 150-pound person burns per hour while doing yard work and home repair, according to the American College of Sports Medicine:

- Refinishing carpentry, caulking, laying or removing carpet, laying tile or linoleum, repairing appliances, painting: 306
- Cleaning gutters, hanging storm windows, painting exterior: 341
- Building a fence, installing rain gutters, using a chain saw, roofing, chopping wood, shoveling snow: 409
- Sawing hardwood: 511

Vacuum Lunge. Turn on the vacuum cleaner and stand in a dirty spot. Hold the vacuum attachment with your left hand. Push the vacuum forward as you take a big step with your right leg. Bend both knees until your left calf is parallel to the floor and your right knee is directly above (not past!) your toes. Pull the vacuum as you return to standing. Switch arms and legs and repeat, moving forward each time. The lunge strengthens and defines your thighs and buttocks. If you move quickly and frequently to other dirty spots, you'll get an aerobic effect—and a clean house faster.

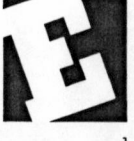

Work the House. Spring or not, dedicate a weekend afternoon or weekday evening at home to a flurry of meaningful, major housecleaning. Turn on some fast-paced, motivating music that makes you want to move, and do those chores you keep putting off. Turn the mattress. Rearrange the furniture. Scrub behind the toilet. Wash windows. Keep the pace of activity in tune with your spirited music, and you'll get your heart rate up, burn calories, and get a tremendous feeling of satisfaction from crossing those chores off your list.

Dirty Dancing. Time to clean house? Turn on some fast music that makes you want to dance and play it loudly enough to be heard over the vacuum cleaner. The music will make you vacuum, sweep, and mop faster, increasing the calories you burn.

Mow, Mow, Mow Your Lawn

Not all lawn mowers are equal. Here's the difference in calories burned by a 150-pound person for 1 hour of mowing the lawn, using different equipment. (Actually, you'll burn even more calories using the hand mower, because it will take longer to get the job done.)

- Using a riding mower: 170
- Using a power mower, walking: 341
- Using a hand mower, walking: 409

254

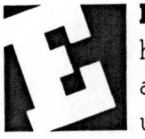 **Housecleaning Calorie Blitz.** In case you think housecleaning is wimpy work, take a look at how fast a 150-pound person burns calories doing 30 minutes of these activities:

- Carpet sweeping, sweeping floor: 112
- Mopping, vacuuming: 119
- Scrubbing floors, bathroom, bathtub: 129
- Sweeping garage or sidewalk: 136
- Moving furniture, carrying boxes: 204
- Moving furniture, carrying boxes upstairs: 306
- Lying on couch watching someone else clean your house: 34

Cardio Study Outdoors. Having trouble justifying leaving your house to exercise because you have a test to study for, a report to prepare, or a manual your boss said you had to read by Monday? Your tape recorder is your new best friend. Read the notes you have to study or brainstorm into the tape recorder. Take that taped info with you into the wilderness, and repeat the information as you listen and hike. Your mind will be more alert so you'll think better and learn faster. And the scenery sure beats the wall in front of your desk. Caution: Although listening to your tape as you walk or run through town might seem like a good idea, it's better to keep your ears and mind alert to the traffic and people around you.

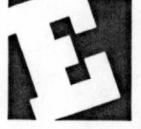

Garden Fitness. You can get yourself and your garden in great shape at the same time. Gardening is immensely satisfying and self-nurturing (even therapeutic), as you get outdoors working in and with the earth. Your toil in the soil results in green growth, beautiful blooms, and edible treats. And, if you grow vegetables, you'll find that homegrown produce is many times tastier than any you can buy, and you'll expend more calories maintaining your garden than you will take in by eating the produce from it. Here are some activities and how many calories per hour a 150-pound person burns from each one:

- Watering (standing or walking): 102
- Picking fruit, vegetables (moderate effort): 204
- Raking lawn, sacking grass and leaves: 272
- Planting, weeding: 306
- Clearing land, hauling branches, digging, spading: 341
- Gardening with heavy power tools, tilling: 409

Cardio Study Indoors. Use the study tape idea from Cardio Study Outdoors, but listen to your study tape with a headset while you work out on any cardio machine at home or at the gym: rower, stair machine, treadmill, elliptical trainer, ski machine, aerobic rider, or exercise bike.

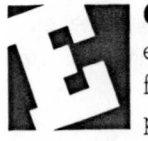 **Clearing House.** Okay, time to get rid of that closetful of clothes that were in style when you graduated from high school (and could fit into them). At a brisk pace, without stopping to think if you'll actually wear that fringed vest or size 5 jeans again, start packing up everything you haven't worn for the past three years or more for your local Goodwill or Salvation Army. Don't stop there: While you're on a roll, pack up all the books and magazines you'll never read or reread to donate to the local library or hospital. Carry everything to the car. Whew, that's a workout. And doesn't it feel good to have some shelf and closet space again? Hint: Deliver everything before you can change your mind.

Speed Reading. Buy (or check out of the library) a book you really want to read. Reserve it for reading *only* when you're walking on the treadmill or some other cardio equipment that leaves your hands free for page turning. Put a reading rack on your favorite cardio machine at home or the gym rather than holding the book. Be careful not to compromise your workout by leaning on the railing of the stair machine or treadmill—stay upright, keep good form, and read on. You'll look forward to your reading time and maybe even stay on the cardio machine longer than you would otherwise.

 **Train Your Tongue.** Learn a language by cassette by playing it on your headset as you walk the park, run the track, or work out on an indoor cardio machine.

Kegel Anytime

Mild urinary stress incontinence—urinary leakage—is a problem encountered by many women during pregnancy, after childbirth, and after menopause, especially when they laugh, sneeze, cough, jump, or exert themselves. Kegel exercises strengthen muscles that control urination by contracting the sphincter muscles of the bladder neck and the vagina.

To "Kegel," simply clench the pelvic muscles, as if you are trying to stop the flow of urine. Try to hold the contraction for 5 seconds or more, and take another 5 seconds to slowly relax. The New York State Office of the American College of Obstetricians and Gynecologists recommends that you do 10- to 20-second Kegels repeated 10 to 20 times in a row, 3 or 4 times a day.

Do your Kegels standing, sitting, and lying down. They're an ideal exercise for when you're doing something else—working, driving, walking, riding a bicycle, traveling in a bus or airplane, doing other exercises, cooking . . . you name it. No one will notice you are doing them. Work up to 5 minutes at a time.

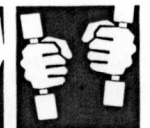**TV Circuit Training.** Work out to your favorite television program. No, you don't have to tune in to some aerobic babe doing leg lifts (unless you want to, of course!). Your favorite medical, court, or crime show will do just fine. Dance, jog, jump rope, or hop on the exercise bike while the program is on. During commercials, drop down for push-ups or crunches on the rug. Combining longer sets of aerobic exercise with short sets of strength training keeps your heart rate elevated even during the strength sets, burning more calories and giving you a stronger cardiovascular effect. Caution: When you're going from an aerobic exercise to one where you're on the floor, keep your head above heart level to avoid dizziness. Drink plenty of water.

Alphabet Thighs. Anytime you have to sit—on the bus, in a movie, at the computer, watching television—do this strengthener for the thighs. Sit up straight and lift one leg so the foot is slightly off the floor. Use your foot to "write" each letter of the alphabet in the air, rotating at the knee. The bigger the letters, the more the thigh muscles work. Advanced: Extend the leg straight to "write" the alphabet, rotating at the hip instead of the knee.

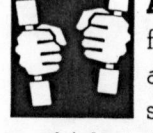 **Alphabet Shoulders.** Here's another strengthener for any time you have to sit or stand (and don't mind attracting attention). Hold your arms straight at shoulder height in front of you and out to the diagonal (about halfway between straight ahead and out to the side). Lower your shoulders and shoulder blades, and keep them lowered throughout the exercise. Use your whole arm to "write" each letter of the alphabet in the air, rotating at the shoulder. You'll look as if you're conducting an orchestra grandly. The bigger the letters, the more the shoulder muscles work.

 **Ride the Rug.** Spin your wheels on the stationary bike as you watch television or read. If you don't have a stationary bike, get a wind trainer (a.k.a. track stand) for your outdoor bike. The back wheel sets on a roller that gives you resistance as you pedal off calories while watching your favorite shows.

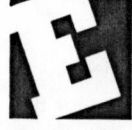 **Get Up and Change.** Hide the remote, and get off your sofa to change channels when you absolutely must watch television. Using the remote to change channels requires less than 1 calorie. Getting up and changing the channel takes 3 calories. Not much, but it adds up if you're a frequent television watcher and a frequent channel-changer.

Tape TV

You can save time by taping your favorite program and watching it later. If you fast-forward through the commercials, you can watch a 60-minute program in 45 minutes. That leaves you 15 minutes to—what else?—exercise!

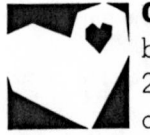 **Get Help.** Buy or rent a motivational audiotape— business, spiritual, or self-help—and listen to it for 20 to 30 minutes while working out on your favorite cardio machine, or take your tape for a walk.

Volunteer Your Body

There's nothing like doing good for others to make you feel good about yourself. Plenty of volunteering activities need physically active people. Contact your local volunteering clearinghouse (or do a computer search on "volunteering opportunities" + your location) to find out about the many opportunities to help your community and get your exercise at the same time. For example, you might do one or more of the following:

- Clean up the local beach or park by sorting recyclables and picking up trash.
- Help dig and plant a community garden.
- Take convalescent-home residents for walks or push them in wheelchairs.
- Sort, pack, deliver, or serve food for your community's food bank.

- Help clean up a creek or weed a native garden.
- Participate in a fundraising walk or bike event for your favorite charity, collecting donations based on the number of miles you walk or bicycle.
- Decorate for special events, like a Chamber of Commerce business fair.
- Be a park rover, walking or hiking the park's trails, trailheads, and beach areas, providing information to visitors about the park's natural, cultural, and historical resources and rules.
- Help out at a local fundraiser by setting up or cleaning up afterward.
- Volunteer with activities at a camp for disadvantaged youth or kids with medical conditions.
- Become a Big Brother or Big Sister, and take your little brother or sister on physically active excursions: walking the zoo or the beach, swimming, ice-skating, roller-skating, building a snowman—no computer games!
- Be a handyman or handywoman for a shut-in, doing repairs, carpentry, or whatever needs doing.
- Lead or assist a trail event, such as a hike or a mountain bike or horseback ride.
- Shelve books at your public library.

(Note that the first six activities are suitable for families. Teaching your child how good it feels to help others can be a rewarding, lifelong lesson.)

12

Appendix

9   **Resources**   3

6

OCCASIONALLY WE'VE MENTIONED HELPFUL FITNESS TOOLS that can either enhance your exercise routine or motivate you to stick with it. Here is more information about these tools, including where to buy them, and other resources we thought you'd find helpful.

Resistance Bands (Dyna-Bands)

Strength training increases your muscles' ability to perform better, increases your metabolic rate so you'll burn more calories   **263** even at rest, and gives you a shapely look. Strength training also helps to maintain or even increase bone density. You can use weights or machines, or get the same benefits at low cost and great convenience with resistance bands made especially for strength training, such as Dyna-Bands, which are stretchy latex strips, 3 feet by 6 inches, that you pull or push to strengthen your muscles. The muscles respond as if you were using weights, as long as you use a difficult enough band. (They're available in four different intensities.)

Read more about Dyna-Bands, including where to order them, at *www.joanprice.com/products/dynabands.htm* or phone 1-888-BFITTER (1-888-234-8837) toll free.

Some tips for using Dyna-Bands:

- To increase resistance, shorten the working part of the band. If you can't get the range of motion you need when you shorten it enough to make the exercise difficult, use a higher intensity band. The harder the resistance—as long as you can keep correct form—the more the muscle will respond by getting stronger.
- How fast? A slow and controlled set of about 6 seconds— 2 seconds up and 4 seconds down—is safe and effective. If you rush, momentum takes over and the muscle you're trying to strengthen does less work and gets less benefit.

- How often? Two or 3 times a week is plenty, spaced evenly over the week. Never strength-train the same muscles 2 days in a row—they need the rest days to get stronger.
- What about form? Focus on the muscle you're strengthening and keep the rest of the body still. Your back should always be neutral—neither rounded nor arched. Breathe through the whole motion, exhaling with the exertion. Be careful to slowly release—never let the band snap back to its original position. Always warm up before and stretch after strength training.
- If the bands snap away when you're trying to anchor them with your feet, the problem is either that you're not pressing your *heel* on the band or that you're letting your heels come up as you perform the movement. Make sure you're anchoring with the heel (not the ball of the foot) and that you keep your body weight firmly over your heels without letting your knees come forward of your toes.
- Care and feeding of Dyna-Bands: Store bands out of direct sunlight in a bag or box, and dust them occasionally with baby powder, talcum powder, or cornstarch to keep them supple. If they get wet, lay them out flat to dry, then powder and store them. Remove rings and other jewelry that could catch on the bands and tear them. If a tear develops, discard the band. (Bands should last for years with proper care.)

Resources

Exercise Videotapes

If you're buying exercise videotapes, don't rely on the few titles available at the local video rental store or library. You'll find a much more extensive and satisfying selection of hundreds of exercise videotapes at Collage Video (1-800-433-6769, *www.collagevideo.com*) and Amazon.com (*www.amazon.com;* under "search" select either DVD or VHS and type in "exercise" or a more specific term like "step" or "yoga"). If you're not sure what to order, start by reading the reviews of recommended videos at *www.joanprice.com/products/videos.htm*. Both Collage and Amazon also have reviews.

Pedometers

Pedometers don't just measure walking, but also dancing, running, climbing stairs—any activity in which you're taking steps. (They don't measure activities like rowing or weightlifting, however.) You're aiming for 10,000 steps a day, which, according to Stanford University and the Cooper Institute for Aerobics Research, yields health benefits. A pedometer makes a game out of getting your daily steps. One reliable and inexpensive pedometer is the New Lifestyles DigiWalker. Clip this tiny (about 1½ × 2 inches), lightweight gizmo to your belt or waistband in the morning, wear it all day, and see how many steps you accumulate over the course of a day. Read more about the DigiWalker, including purchase information, at *www.joanprice.com/prod ucts/ digi.htm.*

How to Track Calories Burned

How did we figure out the calories burned by the activities we mentioned in this book? Here's how we did it, and you can do it yourself with a calculator and some patience. It's a complicated task, but if you'd like the satisfaction of knowing exactly how many calories you burned with all your extra activity, follow these steps:

- Go to *http://prevention.sph.sc.edu/Tools/Compendium _tracking.pdf* and download "The Compendium of Physical Activities Tracking Guide" from the Prevention Research Center at the University of South Carolina. This guide, originally published in *Medicine and Science in Sports and Exercise* from the American College of Sports Medicine, gives the MET values (energy costs) for 1 hour of hundreds of physical activities. Print out all the pages for reference.
- You'll need to know your weight in kilograms (Kg). One pound equals .454 Kg, so multiply your weight in pounds by .454. A 150-pound person weighs 68.1 Kg, for example (150 × .454 = 68.1).
- Next find your activity in the compendium and multiply the

METs by your weight in kilograms. That's how many calories you burn in 1 hour of that activity.

- If you didn't perform the activity for a full hour, figure out how many calories you burned for the duration you performed the activity. Divide by 60 to find the calories per minute, then multiply by the number of minutes. Or, if you did the activity for 15 minutes, just divide by 4 (a quarter of an hour) directly. If you did the activity for 30 minutes, divide by 2 (a half hour).

Here's an example to make this easier. You weigh 200 pounds and you bathed your dog Paws (who wasn't really in the mood for a bath and didn't stand still very well) for 18 minutes. Here's how you would go about figuring out the calories you burned:

1. Find your weight in kilograms: $200 \times .454 = 90.8$ Kg.
2. Find the METs for your activity: Bathing a dog is listed in the Compendium under "home activities (standing, bathing dog)" at 3.5 METs.
3. Multiply $90.8 \times 3.5 = 317.8$ calories burned per hour.
4. Divide 317.8 by $60 = 5.3$ calories burned per minute.
5. Multiply 5.3×18 (the number of minutes it took to wash Paws) $= 95.4$ calories burned getting a clean dog.

(If you wash Paws once a week, that's 4,961 calories burned each year—you'll lose almost 1½ pounds of body fat with just that one activity!)

Now you figure one out!

Your weight in pounds _____ × .454 = _____ , your weight in kilograms.

Description of activity_____.

METs for activity _____.

Multiply your weight in kilograms by the METs for your activity = _____ , the calories you burn doing this activity for 1 hour.

Divide by 60 = _____ , the calories you burn doing this activity for 1 minute.

How many minutes did you perform this activity? _____
Multiplying your answer above by this number = _____ , the calories you burned doing this activity.

Whew!

Youth Fitness

Learn more about how to get your child fit, including specific strengthening and stretching exercises for children and teens, in a 36-page fitness handbook for youth ages 6 to 17 from the President's Council on Physical Fitness and Sports at *www.fitness.gov/getfit.pdf*.

If you have an overweight child, read *The Surgeon General's Call to Action to Prevent and Decrease Overweight and Obesity* at *www.surgeongeneral.gov/topics/obesity/calltoaction/fact_adolescents.htm*.

Author's Web Site

Joan Price invites you to read dozens of free articles about fitness at *www.joanprice.com*. If you've enjoyed this book, please send your comments to Joan at *joan@joanprice.com*.

Index

Index

Printed in the United States
123735LV00004B/2/P

9 780595 514786